Creative Arts
with Older People

Creative Arts
with Older People

Janice McMurray

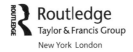

Routledge
Taylor & Francis Group
New York London

First published 1990 by The Haworth Press, Inc.

Published 2017 by Routledge
711 Third Avenue, New York, NY 10017, USA
2 Park Square, Milton Park, Abingdon, Oxon OX14 4RN

Routledge is an imprint of the Taylor & Francis Group, an informa business

Creative Arts with Older People has also been published as *Activities, Adapatation & Aging*, Volume 14, Numbers 1/2 1989.

Library of Congress Cataloging-in-Publication Data

Creative arts with older people / Janice McMurray, author
    p.   cm. – (Activities, adaptation & aging ; v. 14, nos. 1/2)
    Includes bibliographical references.
    ISBN 0-86656-929-4
    1. Handicraft. 2. Aged – Recreation. I. McMurray, Janice. II. Series.
TT157.C716   1990
790.1'926 – dc20   89-20049
                                                                                    CIP

ISBN 13: 978-0-86656-929-3 (hbk)

Creative Arts
with Older People

CONTENTS

ABOUT THE AUTHOR

Janice McMurray, MSW, is the Creative Arts Coordinator at The Hermitage, a retirement community in Richmond, Virginia. A former adult protective service worker for the Social Services Department in Richmond, she received a grant in 1981 from the Virginia Commission for the Arts to do expressive art work with people living in adult homes in the Richmond area. She earned her Master's in Social Work degree from Virginia Commonwealth University, where she also took many studio art classes. She is active in the Richmond art community and is a member of the Richmond Artists' Association.

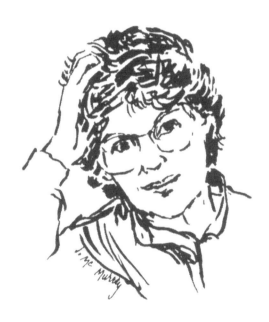

Foreword

This book combines the author's artistic skill, her understanding of the needs of older people, and the use of the creative process as experienced in poetry, music, movement, painting, clay modeling, sculpture, and dramatic expression to enrich the lives of individuals and groups.

It is generally accepted that creative experience can facilitate the expression of ideas and feelings. There are other benefits that can come from increased sensory stimulation such as the development of new skill, improved self esteem, opportunities to relate to others in more meaningful ways, an increased dynamic awareness of self, and heightened responsiveness to the environment. The activities described in this book bring into play perceptual experiences that culminate in finished art products.

The art activities that Janice McMurray describes come from her personal experiences as an artist and as a social worker. They are also based on many years of working with older people. There is respect for her students and artistic integrity in the kinds of activities she has selected. These activities demonstrate her interest in providing opportunities for authentic expressive art experiences.

Janice's knowledge of art materials and her descriptions of art processes are very helpful. The way she has introduced each activity with goals for each activity and the benefits to be derived helps the instructor become aware of the potential within each activity and gives clues to the leader as to how to maximize the experience for the students. Her recommendation for using good quality art materials is an important one in that there is a much better chance to have good quality art work and fewer frustrations in learning how to manipulate the materials. Students can take pride in professional-looking art work. It also reassures them that they are being treated as adults involved in an adult activity.

Her descriptions of how to introduce each activity are helpful for the instructor in the process of motivating the students. One of the important aspects for older people is the opportunity to discuss and develop ideas around a common theme. It enables the group to share their rich and varied experiences in life. It helps prepare them to take the risks involved in using art media for self expression. Once they take up the challenge and experience the pleasure of involvement in using more of their senses, they can experience the reward of having a tangible finished art product.

Those who have guided others through the creative process can relate to what Janice says about how much can be learned from relationships with students and how much it can contribute to the growth and development of the teacher as well as the students for whom this was written.

Charlotte Scotch, ATM, ATR
(Master in Art Therapy,
Registered Art Therapist)

Introduction

The field of gerontology has very little literature that refers to the practice of the expressive arts. In preparing this collection, I have drawn on my own years of experience, including my time since 1981 as creative arts coordinator at The Hermitage Methodist Home in Richmond, Virginia. In this position, I have been able to bring together and use my experience as a practicing artist and my training as a social worker.

My suggestions for working with the elderly are a result of trial and error, and reflect an artist's understanding and appreciation of the creative process, my knowledge of the abilities of the people with whom I was working, and my experience with basic social work theories that had proved successful in my earlier years as a caseworker. My formal education includes a bachelor's degree in art from West Virginia University, a master's in social work from Virginia Commonwealth University, many additional hours in art at VCU and George Washington University, plus the study of art therapy at J. Sargeant Reynolds Community College.

An earlier career as a social worker for the city of Richmond brought me into contact with persons discharged from mental institutions, abused adults and neglected elderly persons. Working with them was stressful, and I turned to art work as an emotional release from my intense involvement in their lives. Ironically, I found that I could not separate myself from my daily experiences. My art work reflected the human drama that I had sought to escape, but apparently could not.

This art work became the basis for my first art show, at the Richmond Public Library in 1974. The show, which portrayed the condition of my clients, included paintings of them (with their permission) and co-workers, and the reconstruction of a kitchen of a typical elderly client. The kitchen was made of old linoleum, wallpaper, chairs and an ironing board taken from houses being torn

1

down in Fulton Bottom, an area of Richmond undergoing urban renewal.

The show was my world and my clients' world and was well received by the public. The Welfare Kitchen traveled around the city on display and eventually was installed permanently in The People Place, a Richmond public schools building visited by schoolchildren to learn how people in other countries and cultures live.

This pouring out of my tensions into art demonstrates how the arts can be used as tools to enable persons to express themselves, recognizing that whatever people produce is an extension of their very beings, and therefore worthwhile. As creative arts coordinator, my job at the Hermitage is to provide opportunities and materials that stimulate creative activity and lead to an enriched life, not necessarily to an attractive product. Residents learn that whatever they do is acceptable and that they will not be judged on their performance. I do not presume to interpret or to analyze the work, but to provide the elderly with opportunities to express themselves in visual terms. An experience thus depicted is made concrete and more readily remembered and learned from.

Those working with older people in art may find that they are not comfortable working with all art forms. Although I am most familiar with the visual arts, I found I could not limit myself to that area alone, but really needed to include all the arts. It's not that I was qualified to cover all areas, but that I saw the need to make available a variety of expressive art forms to reach people who could not express their response to the world by making pictures.

Some persons had such distorted spatial orientation that nothing was gained by painting; these same people could be very imaginative when it came to playing with puppets. Those with strong backgrounds in language learned to speak movingly through poetic images. And there were people with limited memory abilities who derived satisfaction from working within a structured system using step-by-step instructions.

Interaction with students is usually on two levels — psychological and artistic. Even though I am always aware of the therapeutic process and give that priority, I cannot help being enthusiastic over the art pieces my students produce. Again, this doesn't mean giving indiscriminate praise, but seeing and appreciating the individuality of a painting, the special approaches unique to one person.

I find it exciting to recognize the ways in which people perceive their surroundings when given the freedom to execute an art challenge in a personal style. When we create we feel alive, we feel effective, and we know that we are significant.

An account in Bruno Bettleheim's book *The Informed Heart* bears this out. Jewish prisoners in a concentration camp were marching lifelessly to the gas chambers without resisting when a sadistic SS officer singled out one of the group, a blank-faced woman who used to be a dancer. He ordered her to dance for him. "She did and as she danced, she approached him, seized his gun, and shot him down. She too was immediately shot to death."[1]

Dr. Bettleheim surmises that "dancing made her once again a person. Dancing, she was singled out as an individual . . . no longer was she a number, a nameless, depersonalized prisoner, but the dancer she used to be. Transformed, however momentarily, she responded like her old self, destroying the enemy bent on her destruction, even if she had to die in the process."[2]

In January 1981, I received a grant from the Virginia Commission of the Arts to do expressive art work in a number of adult homes in Richmond. The goal was to enhance the quality of life for adults who needed supervision and who had little motivation to pursue any activities. Meeting with them weekly, I used whatever art forms and techniques I could find that would elicit positive responses. Sometimes it was music, sometimes dancing, sometimes painting.

My bean bag animals and large dancing dolls fulfilled more than one function. Besides their use in promoting play, they allowed residents to show affection and to imagine the animals and dolls were real. A blind man held an almost life size rag doll, dancing with her to music that I played on a tape recorder. (He named her Bertha after an old girl friend.) Watching them, I realized that he loved dancing and that more activities along this line would have benefited him.

On one occasion Bertha disappeared, and I found her in the room of an elderly woman who had run off with her, hiding the doll in her bed. Seeing the adults' need for someone to love, I wished I could

have provided each person with his or her own huggable companion. When a tough-talking young ex-offender became attached to a
little soft, brown monkey I used in a game, it became apparent he
needed it more than I did, so I let him keep it.

Almost everyone in adult homes responds to music. Persons with
memory problems have a repertoire of songs they learned when
they were young. Many remember hymns. Retarded people who
can't read know the words to countless songs. At each home where
I worked there invariably was someone who could carry a tune and
be enlisted to help lead the singing. When I learned what songs that
person could sing, I often had copies made for the group.

I remember particularly a sad man with an alcohol problem who
had been at one time a member of a barber shop quartet. Although
he hadn't sung in years, he had a wonderful, deep voice. Because
he had performed publicly, I asked if he would mind singing certain
verses alone while the rest of the group came in on the chorus as a
sort of "backup" group. He agreed, and the result was so thrilling
that I taped the group's rendition of "Love Lifted Me" and "Down
by the Old Mill Stream."

The second song lent itself to illustrations, so we divided it into a
dozen scenes with several people drawing their versions of the old
mill and a stream. Clear acetate was placed over the drawings and
with water-soluble projector pens, each drawing was traced to be
used with an overhead projector. After putting them into an appropriate sequence we showed them on the wall accompanied by the
tape recording of "Down by the Old Mill Stream."

In my work with the adult home residents I attempted to identify
their strengths and adapt my program to develop those strengths.
However, I was the main beneficiary of the experience in terms of
learning and research, and the residents needed far more than I
could give them in weekly one-hour sessions.

Soon after my city-wide work was over, I was offered an opportunity to do similar expressive art activities with residents at the
Hermitage Methodist Home in Richmond. I accepted the job because it was a church-related adult home and health-care center and
I never had worked in that kind of environment before. Incorporat-
ing religious beliefs with art work and social work would bring
together the three most important areas of my life.

The Hermitage residents have the basic needs of their life met: food, shelter and secure surroundings. They are likely to suffer from serious health problems and the limitations of advanced age. And because they live in a church-related facility sharing a common bond of religious faith, I am now able to draw on that background extensively for art activities.

My goal is to help residents express themselves creatively, and to maintain and realize their own unique identities. For example, a person may choose to work with a puppet allowing that puppet to speak the person's inner thoughts. Abilities and imagination never called upon until now are thus revealed.

In childhood, many persons' creative attempts were judged against academic standards having nothing to do with their own personal experiences. Their teachers praised students who could draw objects realistically. Children for whom this expectation was impossible usually gave up and assumed that art was not for them. When people are freed of this stereotype, they begin to grow and blossom in their art classes. It has been rewarding for me to watch this happen and to observe the pride and satisfaction as residents become aware that from within themselves they have created something original, something of value.

Equally significant is the relationship between art teacher and pupil. Unless a level of trust has been established between them, revealing one's self through one's art work is difficult for the pupil because it involves taking a risk.

As their leader, I always try to convey care and empathy for the feelings of the class members. What they experience emotionally takes precedence over the craft or art work being done. To create an atmosphere of safety, I make clear that the ground rules include respect for each other and each other's work. Competition has no place in this setting of mutual acceptance, equal time to be heard, and freedom to follow one's inclinations.

The art sessions described in this book have been held primarily with Hermitage Methodist Home residents who need physical help or supervision: those in the Health Care Center and the Personal Care Unit. As the creative arts coordinator, I have also been responsible for art activities with active residents, many of whom want to improve their artistic skills. I believe that everyone can draw and paint. If residents want to develop their personal styles, they certainly can, and I am glad to help them.

As a result of the classes, our residents were invited to show their watercolors on three occasions at the Richmond Public Library. I don't encourage comparison or competition, but I think it is appropriate to show what one has done and to take pleasure in it. Many requests to buy the art work came when the public viewed the shows. But few of the artists were willing to part with their paintings for financial gain. They preferred to give them to their children or other relatives, or to keep them in their rooms.

Slides made of the residents' art work can be made to enjoy it again later. Art slide shows with music accompaniment are also enjoyable for relatives to watch.

Because our art program has been designed to meet the needs of the residents living at the Hermitage, it is stronger in some areas than others. Then too, the residents have selected subjects and crafts I would not have been inclined to choose, but that turned out to be successful adventures — ceramics and basket making, for example. We have covered much territory in my six years at the Hermitage and our experiences may be useful to others in similar situations.

The following pages describe and give directions for some of the art activities and projects we have found rewarding creatively, psychologically, and socially.

Finger Painting

Goal: To provide an opportunity for people to use imagination, express feelings.

Benefits of medium: Reduction of inhibitions about art activity as paint is used in a loose, flowing manner with the hand as the art tool.

Materials:

- Large brushes
- Container of water
- Large sheets finger painting paper, table space for large paper
- 5 jars of color (red, blue, green, yellow, black)
- 5 teaspoons (one for each color)
- Aprons, basin of water and paper towels for washing hands

When I introduce finger painting to groups who have not done it before, or even groups who have, I can expect them to be slightly resistant. They think this type of painting is for children. Since it's messy, they're reluctant to put their hands directly into the paint.

I like to tell them about my friend, a finger painter who has had one-woman shows of her work at respected places. She works in this medium because it is very expressive. There is no reason such a good tactile experience should be limited to children. We sometimes forget the pleasurable sensations it affords to handle the material directly rather than through an intermediate object such as a brush.

First I demonstrate to the group how to use the materials. Starting with a large sheet of smooth finger-paint paper, I point out its shiny surface and wet it with a large brush. Next I drop a spoonful of finger paint onto the surface and begin manipulating it with my fingers until the strokes or smears begin to remind me of something.

I use large motions so that those watching will be influenced to do the same. These broad movements will help them become less inhibited. After I add a spoonful of another color, the painting should start to resemble something meaningful to me which can be given a name — a fanciful name perhaps.

Although it isn't necessary to the process, I have found that music helps to loosen one's thoughts and inspire visual images. Pastoral music such as Smetana's "The Moldau" or lively themes from musicals like "Cabaret" can set the mood. I have also used an environmental cassette called "Ultimate Thunder."[1]

When people first experience finger painting, they may be hesitant. But they soon begin to lose their inhibitions and enjoy the possibilities in simple movements that spread the finger paint across the paper. There should be several colors of paint available from which to choose. The colors the people select will often dictate the mood of their painting, which may not reflect their own mood at the beginning of the session. Usually there is a lot of laughing and commenting about what is beginning to appear in their paintings.

I ask each participant to give his or her picture an identity by naming and dating it. Finger painting is different from other painting experiences in that it reflects more directly how a person feels at the time.

A resident who had Parkinson's disease and could not speak was able to use this medium fairly well, especially with a friend. She could be a part of this painting group even though she wasn't able to participate in any others. Although the rest of us were not always sure what she was trying to say in her paintings, it was clear she saw something meaningful in them.

These kinds of paintings are never put up for permanent display as they are an end in themselves. The focus is the painter's process, not the end result in terms of "art." Residents not involved in painting frequently regard such efforts as childish and may not understand what is in the paintings nor appreciate the feelings that may have evolved during the process. Their comments could unintentionally ridicule and hurt the painter.

At the end of the class we might have a brief time for members to share what came out of their paintings. I tape the pictures to the wall of the workshop with masking tape so we can view our efforts for a few minutes and read the titles. If a person is unable to say anything, I may comment on what I see in a picture or what I observed or heard as the painting was going on.

How to Paint a Rainbow for People Who Have Never Painted with Watercolors

Goals: To provide an opportunity for people to have a successful painting experience. The products will reflect individuals' perception and color preferences. Appropriate for both mentally capable and mentally limited persons.

Materials: (For each participant)

- 9" × 12" watercolor paper
- Box of paints (preferably with 16 colors)
- Baby food jar filled with water
- Brush (size 5)
- Paper towels (for mopping up excess water and creating interesting effects)

We use baby food jars as water containers because they are less likely to be knocked over than plastic cups. We keep a supply of paper towels on hand as blotters for removing excess water. (Paper towels should be soft, not the harsh brown type.) Applying towels to the surface creates stains and variations in color that otherwise would not be achieved. Our people have learned to work with brush in the one hand and towel in the other.

Watercolor painting is a poetic medium in that it evokes a mood, the colors are light and airy, and the images are often suggested rather than clearly defined. Our residents accept it since water colors are recognized as an adult medium. When applied to rough paper they can be manipulated in many different ways with a brush and are ideal for painting a rainbow with a washy effect using a "wet on wet" technique. It is important to remember that the colors tend to pale as they dry.

To prepare a group in the Health Care Unit to paint a rainbow, we listen to a recording of "Somewhere Over the Rainbow." Then we talk about the promise of the rainbow, how God set it in the clouds as a symbol that the earth would never again be covered with water. As a reinforcement of the significance of the rainbow, I may read aloud the Scriptural reference in Genesis 9:12-18. Then we name the colors of the rainbow — red, orange, yellow, green, blue, indigo and violet.

Each person is given a piece of watercolor paper (about 9" × 12"), which can be taped to the table with masking tape if students have limited hand capability or are weak. I believe it is important to use real watercolor paper, even though it is expensive, and a fairly decent brush. (This is how we use money we make at our annual bazaar.) Ordering paper from an art store catalog in quantity and cutting it into smaller portions decreases the cost.

Each student is also given a water container, brush and box of colors along with a pencil and paper towels. I ask them to take their pencils and draw the bands of color of the rainbow in an arc over a horizon line. Even though we have counted seven colors, they generally draw only four or five bands.

The next step is to fill in the sky with paint. The sky area should be moistened with a brush using clear water, leaving the area of the rainbow dry. The brush should be loaded heavily with blue paint (choosing among three blues in a box of 16 colors). Beginning at the top left corner, making strokes from left to right, the participant should work his way down the paper. If the brush needs more paint, he should add more, dipping the brush in water first.

The usual way of filling in the sky is to have the deepest color at the top, gradually fading to a pale color at the horizon line. No one is required to do this, but it is helpful to know how to put sky in a picture and suggest distance. The sky closest to us, overhead, is the top part of the picture and the brightest. Objects far away begin to fade as does the sky that is farthest from us. Of course it's all an illusion, and one can do anything one wants to and still create a pleasing picture.

The brush is cleaned after the sky is dry, and the bands of color can be painted in. Unlike the process of painting the sky, the bands of colors for the rainbow are not allowed to dry before the next band is applied. It is necessary to clean the brush only between colors. The colors bleeding onto each other create a lovely effect. No two paintings will be alike and everyone will have a painting with which he or she can be pleased. We have always gotten a good response from outsiders who have seen our rainbows. Two of the rainbows were used as the background against which names of participants in our slide show "The Rainswept Sky" were photographed.

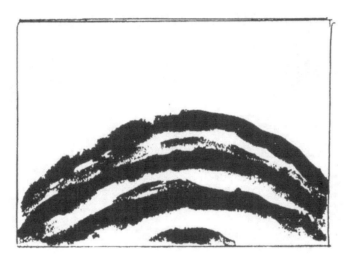

Wet on Wet Rainbow Drawing

Painting Trees
in the Health Care Center

Goal: To teach people how to paint a tree with water colors.

Benefit: Cultural life enriched by an art experience focusing on trees.

Materials: (For each participant)
- 9" × 12" watercolor paper
- Box of paints (preferably with 16 colors)
- Baby food jar filled with water
- Brush (size 5)
- Paper towels (for mopping up excess water and creating interesting effects)
- Sponges (real, not artificial)

Prior to this two—session activity I had drawn the basic skeletal shapes of various trees on large sheets of newsprint. These I taped on the walls around the room. (It is helpful to use an opaque projector, if you have access to one, to enlarge the size of the tree forms.)

At the beginning of the first session we identify the trees by their shapes, some of which are more familiar to the residents than others. Then we talk about various connections they might make with trees—climbing them, sitting in their shade, picking their fruits, swinging in them, cutting them down at Christmastime.

I remind the group that trees are plants grown large. Unlike plants, trees never stop growing, and they don't die at the end of the season. Trees look different under different conditions: from a distance only the general shape is observable with leaves blurred together and colors muted. In the rain, tree trunks look black as they contrast with the color of yellow leaves; in the mist they are shadowy and delicate.

15

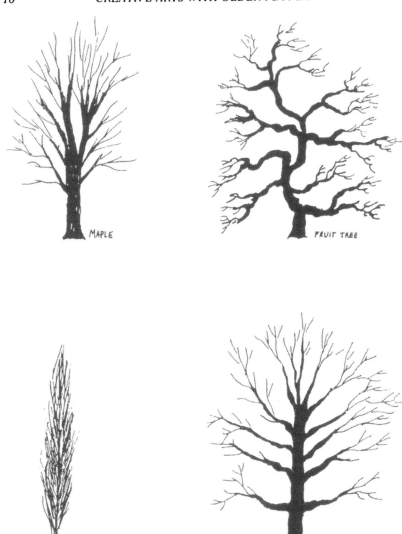

Four Trees

Artists have used many painting techniques to try to convey how trees appear to them. I show details in the jungle paintings of Henri Rousseau's trees, Peter Breughel's forests, Monet's poplars, Seurat's trees made of dots of colors, and Van Gogh's twisted trunks. Since the paintings are varied but pleasing in different ways, the group begins to understand that there is no one best technique for painting trees.

On one occasion as we looked at the works, a woman felt inspired to sing, "I Think That I Shall Never See a Poem Lovely as a Tree." Since I am not a singer, I hummed along with her for support, and someone else whistled as others joined in.

Each person is given a box of watercolors (16 — cake size), a brush, a water container and a piece of basic watercolor paper. (People with the use of only one hand will need their paper taped to the table.) Small genuine sponges make a good texture for simulating leaves.

Next I briefly demonstrate the use of watercolors: dipping the brush in water, tapping off the excess on the side of the jar, twirling the brush around on the cake of watercolor until it is heavily loaded with color, then beginning to paint the trunk of the tree. (It is a good idea to practice beforehand until you have enough control of the medium to feel comfortable with it.) I always paint with a brush in one hand and a paper towel in the other. In this way I can blot the paint from time to time to achieve variations on the painting surface.

I bring in color photographs of trees for the class to work from if they have no tree in mind. I emphasize that a tree is not one color but three — dark green, medium green and light green (if green happens to be the dominant color of their tree). To achieve those three variations they will have to add other colors to their basic hue.

Halfway through their painting people may ask, "What color must I use now?" I tell them what will happen if they add yellow or purple or blue, but I make no suggestions. Older people often have a yellow film over the lens of their eyes which makes blues look like green and distorts other colors also.

For the second session, I place small branches from various trees and bushes in vases and containers on the tables. I suggest the group pretend the branches are to be trees as they paint them. Before they begin, I review ideas from the last session and again show artists' treatment of trees.

As people paint, they tend to converse. Once a woman confined to a geriatric chair remarked how sad it was to see an old tree broken in the field. "Poor old tree lying in the field—you did your best for us, and we haven't even given you decent recognition." Her words seemed to reflect how she might have felt about herself. Then she added that lots of people think trees can read your mind.

One particular group met again with me on the day they had completed their second painting. I displayed for them the two tree paintings they had finished and asked them to look at their results, remembering special trees they had known. When a particular tree came to mind, they could speak to the tree about how they felt about it, and write down their thoughts. Here are some of the poems written by members of the group.

MY TREE

How beautiful you are, my tree!
Often your shade was a welcome to me as I came home.
I loved the days my granddad bored a place in your bark
And put in a spout to let out your sweet sap.
One winter's day we used your fallen leaves
To make a warm nest for our collie to keep warm.
In the spring we watched eagerly for your branches
To show early colors of the dawning spring.
Dear maple of my childhood days,
Do not leave this spot.
I could not bear to see the familiar house
If you were not there.

—Alma Lowance

LOCUST TREE

The rainswept sky
Dropped tears
Upon my locust tree.

—Alma Lowance

PEAR TREE

A sturdy little pear tree
Stood in the far end of the garden in my childhood
And a tomboyish brown-eyed girl chose it
For an imaginary playhouse.
Your leaves, little tree, were smooth
And grew luxuriously.
Sometimes you had small delicious pears
Which were shared by blue jays and catbirds
As well as by my sisters and me.
When I wanted solitude
You afforded me sanctuary.
There among your limbs
I dreamed my childish dreams
Uninterrupted and undisturbed.

—*Kathleen Elmore*

OAK TREE

Dear oak tree, I remember you with pleasure
And the picnics we had under your branches!
Mother and Dad seemed to enjoy it as much as we children
As we watched the squirrels storing acorns
In the crevices of your trunk.
Whenever I see an oak tree
Pleasant memories come to mind.

—*Jo Winton*

Working in Clay

Goal: To create an environment that nurtures imagination; to acquaint the class with techniques of making clay sculpture.

Materials:

- "The Forms of Life" (movie)
- 25 lbs. of clay
- Plastic tablecloth
- Towels or aprons to protect clothing
- Basin of water
- Jars of water
- Paper towels
- Cutting wire to divide the clay
- Simple wooden or plastic modeling tools (tongue depressors and toothpicks are excellent) unless you have future plans to continue working with clay and may want to invest in more professional tools
- Samples of sculpture to handle (I used alabaster carved birds, an African head of ebony, wooden elephants, clay pieces, as many examples of materials as I could find)
- Library books showing well-known pieces of sculpture

Our unit on clay covered six sessions. After first showing a movie, "The Forms of Life," I inquired what sort of sculpture appealed to members of the group. I asked if there were statues with which they were familiar, or if they had ever collected three dimensional objects such as birds, dogs, or dolls. Their lack of response made me feel that sculpture was almost a foreign word to the group.

Trying to convey another way of thinking about sculpture, I picked up a woman's walker and set it on the piano bench. I pointed out that I had taken the walker out of its usual context and put it in a different environment. We could now look at it as a piece of art.

21

It was three-dimensional, had smooth curves, and combined more than one material (rubber, cloth and shiny steel tubing). I mentioned artists who had used cars or wrecks of scrap metal or gilded bicycles. Even Picasso made a goat out of handle bars and pieces of machinery.

When spectators see something ordinary placed on a pedestal in a museum, they are forced to look at in a different way, to think something different, suddenly to see it as unique. Although the class could not reach the level of accepting "junk as art," they at least began to broaden their understanding of what they could create that would be acceptable to me and themselves.

At the second session we had our usual loosening up exercises to a song called "My Aunt Came Back," with lots of body movements. Then we gathered around a plastic-cloth-covered table where everyone was given a lump of clay to experiment with. They were asked to push it, pull it and manipulate it until it started to look like something to them. Then they could begin to develop a form or an image.

At that session they did not "see" much in the clay, so we made pinch pots instead. This was done by inserting both thumbs in the middle of a ball of clay and hollowing it out. The sides were pinched to the desired thickness and the cracks smoothed with water. Designs were made on the sides with toothpicks or screwdrivers — anything that would cause an impression.

We also made hand-built pots. After clay had been rolled into a small ball it was flattened into a round, cookie shape. With both hands the participants rolled another lump of clay into a long snake-like coil. They wound the coil around the edge of the cookie in pinwheel fashion to form the sides of a bowl or pot. More than one coil was needed. These were smoothed together with the hands or a wooden tool like a tongue depressor. Again, texture was added to the surface by imprinting it with sticks, spoon handles or anything that makes an impression on the clay surface.

Another interesting way the group worked with the coil sides was to retain the coil shape. They left small open spaces outside, but the inside of the coils had to be smoothed together to prevent their coming apart when fired in a kiln. Scoring the surfaces that touch

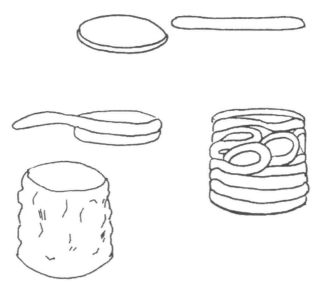

Clay Pots and Tools

each other and adding a bit of water also ensured their melding together.

The third session was devoted to another discussion of art appreciation. In books on sculpture, I showed the group pictures of primitive stylized animals and figures, Easter Island heads, Stonehenge examples, and statues from a park several people had visited in the past. In addition, I showed work from different countries to emphasize the universality of interest in three dimensional objects.

At our fourth session a friend who works in clay came to help us, offering her techniques and giving individual help to residents who could not manage the clay by themselves.

For the fifth session I wanted everyone to have success in making a bird. As a warm-up exercise we imagined we were birds. With eyes closed we spread our wings as widely as possible, swooping and gliding like an eagle, then climbing again to mountain peaks, stopping a while to perch on a limb and rest, then flapping rapidly like a tiny hummingbird darting from flower to flower, preening ourselves, tucking our heads under a wing, taking off bravely to soar over the ocean, flying home again over the treetops, identifying trees as we passed, then setting down safely into our cozy nest. I encouraged people with the use of only one arm to try some motion, even if it was only one hand or the fingers.

A recording we used in that session was John Denver's "I Am the Eagle." It has a nice line: "All those who see me, and all who believe in me share in the freedom I feel when I fly."⁴

Now the participants were ready to make a simple bird. After rolling the clay, into a sausage, they refined and shaped it until one end had a little turned up tail and the other a pointed beak. Two triangles were attached to the sides of the body for wings.

Once the class got the hang of it, they made any number of birds and then began to change the shapes to suit themselves. In a week the birds were ready to be fired in a kiln and painted with ceramic stain. If no kiln had been available, the birds could have been made out of Sculpy, baked in an ordinary oven and painted with acrylic paint. Sculpy is a clay-like medium that does not have to be fired and that will harden when baked. It is rather expensive, so it is more appropriate for small birds than for larger pieces of sculpture.

As we worked, one woman sang "If I Had the Wings of an Angel." (I had never heard her sing by herself before.) Another woman thought her bird looked more like a flying fish so someone began the song, "On the Road to Mandalay, Where the Flying Fishes Play," and many people joined in on that one. I have observed that participants often sing spontaneously when they are working as a group on projects not requiring much concentration.

At the final session I gave the participants a larger chunk of clay than they had used previously, and encouraged them to manipulate it and turn it into whatever occurred to them. Working with a large

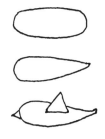

Clay Bird in Development

lump of clay proved to be more difficult than with a small lump since it required more strength in their hands. One woman who had had several strokes and could barely sign her name on a birthday card worked her clay into "a little thing hobbling along" (her title) which I felt was significant. Another fashioned a madonna and child, a common theme among women using this art form.

After the six sessions were over, I placed some of their pieces against a brown velvet cloth in the main display showcase at the Hermitage. Included was a vine nest made by another patient for one of the birds. Almost immediately, to my surprise, a visitor asked to buy it. This is no criterion of success, but it certainly was an indication that the patients need not feel embarrassed by their creations.

I always ask permission to display any work. If people don't want their things shown, of course their wishes are honored. I also have a release form to be signed by individuals if I show their work outside the Hermitage.

Pocket Babies

Goal: Encourage residents' independence by offering them the chance to do something for others.

Benefits of medium: Opportunity to handle various textures and to hold and cuddle soft stuffed dolls.

Materials:

- Bag of polyester Fiberfill
- Yarn (yellow and brown)
- Calico material
- Elmer's glue
- Needle and thread
- Cardboard
- Fabric crayons (Pentel)
- Scissors

About two months before Christmas a few years ago, our Health Care Center activity director asked me if there was something we could do for people in the community. Our residents were forever on the receiving end of gift giving, which increased their feelings of dependency. Couldn't we think of some way to give gifts in return?

We did. The residents and I came up with the idea of pocket babies as gifts for the children at the Crippled Children's Hospital. Here is how this three-session project evolved.

A friend of mine has an extensive collection of old dolls, toys and stuffed animals. When I asked her if she could bring a table's worth to the Health Care Center for people to look at and hold in their arms, she readily agreed. We knew the residents would enjoy looking at worn toys from another era since we had held similar exhibits before. My friend brought teddy bears and dolls that were not too valuable for residents to handle. It was pleasant for them to be re-

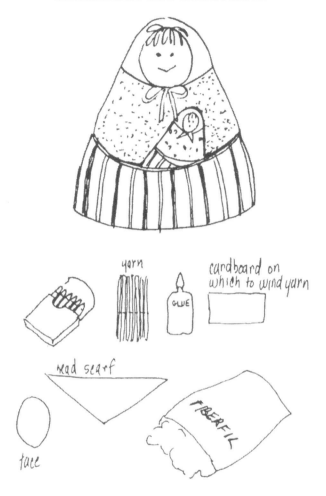

Pocket Baby and Materials

minded of the old days when they had played with similar dolls and toys, and the group spent considerable time holding and cuddling them.

Later I played a Peter, Paul and Mary' recording about childhood games like "Hide and Seek," "Rain, Rain, Go Away," and other songs with children as the focus. I asked people to mention favorite toys and games from their childhood.

As I listened, I noticed a pattern to their stories: almost everyone mentioned a secret spot where he or she had enjoyed playing, a hiding place remembered fondly. (Eyes were closed as they thought of the special places where they had played as children.) One person recalled an attic corner, one a playhouse, another a basement. Two people had actually had tree houses.

With this information in mind, I looked for some type of toy with a secret compartment. After some searching I found a simple, pillow-like doll with an "apron pouch" where something could be hidden. She looked like a peasant, and in her apron she carried a smaller version of herself. In the second doll's apron was an even tinier doll.

I made a sample of the dolls and brought them to the Health Care Center for the group to see. They thought children would like them, and they agreed to make a dozen for the boys and girls at the hospital. It would have been nice for everyone to have made the large mama doll or the tiny baby, but we had time to make only one so we opted for the middle-sized doll with a note hidden in her pocket. I suggest making the largest doll as I think it would be easier.

Because of the physical limitations of the Health Care Center residents, I sewed 12 basic unstuffed bodies from brightly colored calico prints with aprons of contrasting solid colors. Each person chose the color doll she wanted and was given a muslin circle for the face, yarn for hair, Fiberfill stuffing, and a piece of 1/2-inch dowel rod with which to push the stuffing into the doll. Fabric crayons and bottles of Elmer's glue were shared.

Each resident drew eyes, mouth and cheeks on her doll's face with fabric crayon and then glued it on the top part of the triangle body. They glued on yarn for bangs of hair, but bangs could have been painted on instead. Finally, they tied a triangle of cloth around the doll's head, babushka style, and tacked it down. One woman, who could sew well, whipstitched the openings in the dolls after they were stuffed. Then we sat in a circle around the table and shared ideas about messages to be put in the babies' apron pockets: everything from "God bless you" to nursery rhymes was suggested.

When the dolls were finished, they looked so charming that I put them on display in the main showcase at the Hermitage with an explanation that they would be on their way to the Crippled Children's Hospital in time for Christmas. The residents of the Health Care Center appeared pleased with the gifts they had created to bring joy to others.

Fish Printing

Goals: To produce a pleasurable sensory experience by bringing participants into contact with objects of nature.

To increase appreciation of an art technique from another culture.

Benefits of medium: Printing technique is simple to manipulate successfully for those with limited physical or mental abilities.

Materials:

- One or two fresh fish with distinct scales (each fish can be used up to 10 times)
- Wooden board
- Toothpicks
- Small amount of modeling clay
- Two tubes of Speedball printing ink (water soluble)
- Large oil painting brush
- Small oil painting brush
- Paper toweling
- Basin of water
- Paper towels
- Aprons

Fish printing, an old art form from Japan, is different from the usual mode of printing and a great deal of fun to do.

After washing the fish to take off mucus still clinging to its body, I patted it dry, then walked around the group with the fish so that everybody got a chance to admire it at close range and to smell it.

Next I placed the fish on the board using clay to prop up the tail and the fins. (The fish needs to be propped up so that all parts of the

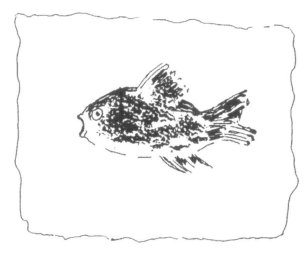

Fish Painting

body are level for printing.) I broke a toothpick in half to keep the mouth open.

Dipping the brush in ink, I applied a thin coat of ink with strokes going with the scales from the head to the tail. After the fish had been painted, I applied one more stroke of paint, this time against the scales from tail to head. I painted the rim of eye but not the eyeball.

Now the residents were ready to print. They laid paper toweling (used because it is soft and simulates the scaled texture of the fish) on the fish and patted it thoroughly until they thought they had a complete impression. Carefully pulling the toweling up, they had an exact replica of the fish with the exception of the eye. The round rim was definite however. With a small brush they painted the circle in another color for dramatic effect.

After deckling the edge of the paper and mounting the fish print on a piece of construction paper with rubber cement, they each had a piece of art work that anyone would be proud of.

Health Care Center residents as well as confused patients can do this activity since it requires no abstract thinking and success is assured. The experience of seeing and smelling a real fish stimulates other senses as well.

At the next session which happened to be in the afternoon, while we still had the fish, we wrote poems, imagining where the fish had been and what its life had been like. We spoke directly to the fish, asking it questions and describing its beauty. The resulting poems were personal and lively.

Key Cats

Goal: To have hands-on experience with new materials (wood, sandpaper, Gesso, polymer gloss) in producing a "folk art" product.

Materials needed for 12 cats:

- Enough 1/4″ plywood for 12 cat silhouettes, approximately 6″ × 10″ in size (to be cut out by the leader)
- Sandpaper
- Newspapers
- Water containers
- Brushes
- Acrylic paint—black, white, orange, pink, green
- Gesso (or white acrylic paint)
- 36 cup hooks (3 for the front of each cat)
- 12 picture hooks (for the back of the cats)
- Aprons
- Paper towels

This four-session activity began with an introduction to folk art. In the room I placed three antique art pieces: a weather vane, an old doll and a quilt. Showing examples from magazines like *Country Living*, *Craft Magazine* and *Home Decorating* I spoke of the resurgence of the appeal of early American objects and art. We also looked at photographs of painted cats on fireplace screens or displayed beside the fireplace. Encouraged to comment on what they liked, the group said the fireplace cats were very colorful.

After reading Edward Lear's poem "The Owl and the Pussycat," I had them do cat stretching exercises. One of our volunteers and I went around the group rubbing each person's back as if stroking a cat. One resident tried to meow like a cat and another person made purring sounds.

35

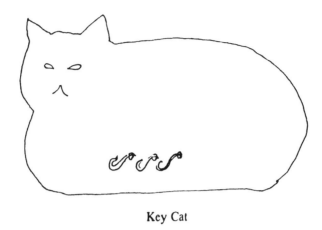

Key Cat

First session: Using a coping saw, I had cut silhouettes of cats out of 1/4″ plywood. (If I hadn't been able to cut the cats from plywood myself, I would have made a pattern and asked the maintenance department or a volunteer to cut them out for me.) The group needed to sand the silhouettes on the edges and give them a coat of white Gesso (white acrylic paint may be substituted) before painting them like folk art cats.

Second session: Members of the class got down to serious work painting their cats. They all chose the kind of cat they wanted to paint, from pictures in magazines or from memory. When people needed assistance with the drawing of ears or mouth, I helped only if they appeared frustrated and likely to give up. I prefer not to make any marks on my students' work, because I want to help them see that anything they do is as valid as anything I might do.

When the instructor draws for the students, it robs them of self-confidence and acceptance of their own work. It's better to provide a model to go by. I prefer to ask questions ("What shape does an ear have?") or suggest they draw a shape in the air first. Acrylic paints dried quickly, and as the last step for that day, the participants put one coat of polymer gloss on the painted cats.

Third session: The class members pounded hanging-type hooks into the backs of the cats so they could be hung on the wall. Cup hooks were screwed to the lower front of the cats so keys could be hung from them. Some of the residents needed a little help, because they lacked sufficient strength. The students ultimately gave most of the cats to their families.

Fourth session: Class members were asked to look at their cats, give them names and have them speak. What did the cats have to say about themselves? What did they like to do? Here are some examples of what my students said:

PATCHES, THE CAT

Patches, the cat, watches the movement in the alley.
His enemies are hiding, awaiting Patches'
Morning walk along the hedges.
He avoids the silly cat wearing the red ribbon
Because he is a fighter.
Gray cats along green hedges
Are not too visible, he decides,
As he stretches out a paw toward the red brick street.
Suddenly a bird flashes by,
Patches darts to his left.
One alarmed chirp. . . . .
The bird is no more.

—Alma Lowance

SALLY, THE SIAMESE

My name is Sally, I'm a Siamese.
When I was ousted from my home
I ran into trouble.
A big horrid dog caught me by the neck.
I think he broke my neck,
I have to hold it one-sided.
I love Bill,
And I sleep on his bed at night.
He is a boy. He is my friend.

—Kathleen Elmore

Displays and Banners

DISPLAYS

Goal: To enhance the residents' environment.

Since health-care and personal care residents often choose to sit and stare at their surroundings, areas where they spend much of their time need frequent changing of visual stimulation. Changing bulletin boards and display walls regularly engenders a feeling of liveliness, a suggestion that "things are happening." An attractive display is upbeat and positive. In contrast, when old floral bouquets (usually from a funeral) droop limply, poinsettias are left to fade and die, Fourth of July decorations remain up in September, the message communicated is one of defeat and neglect.

There are residents who resist taking part in activities but who respond to what they notice in display areas. Observant relatives and friends also get a positive feeling when they visit and realize that the center is a humane place to be.

Displaying and arranging attractive visual items requires planning and time. If the art therapist concentrates solely on the residents' personal expressive experiences, it is easy to neglect doing anything about bulletin boards. Yet the job of creating a visually stimulating environment needs attention too and is well worth doing. In a setting where patients are surrounded by institutional furniture and hospital paraphernalia, any personal touch is noticed at once.

I remember going to an adult home one Christmas season prepared to help them make a crèche. I had brought along all the materials to make the little figures from cloth, starch and clothespins. About five residents were sitting with me at a table when we discovered I had brought nothing to use for the head of the baby in the manger. One of the women spoke up, "I think I have something in my room we can use. A visitor who came to see me dropped some beads from her purse, and I found one after she had gone. It's in my drawer — I'll go get it." She hurried off and was soon back with the precious bead.

In contrast, I thought of my own home with five children and how little attention I pay to our clutter of possessions, let alone one small bead. I was impressed with the simplicity of this woman's world and the notice she took of any change within it.

BANNERS

Goal: To enhance the surroundings by producing one art piece through cooperative group efforts; to heighten the residents' feelings of self-worth and to reflect personal preferences.

One project we do as a cooperative group effort is to make banners for special occasions. If the banner is made in a health care center, people's disabilities must be taken into consideration so that everyone does the things she or he is capable of.

Making a Peace Banner

The day before our art class met in the Health Care Center, I had taken part in a two mile Memorial Day peace march to the Virginia State Capitol in Richmond. I told the class about the experience and included other relevant information — that George Washington had wanted a Department of Peace in addition to a War Department in his cabinet but was unable to achieve the goal; that there was currently a bill before the U.S. Congress to create an Academy for Peace.

This led to a discussion of how difficult it is to resolve disagreements between individuals, much less nations. One woman told how her two sons fought as children. The older boy was "sly" and could "outfox" the younger one. When the second son tried to hit his older brother, Mrs. M. would say, "I know you're angry, but you mustn't kill him." Another resident, Miss J., mentioned someone whose telephone discourtesy always made her angry.

What can people do when they have differences of opinions? We discussed the possibilities, and the group agreed that talking things out is the answer. I asked the students if they would be willing to make a peace banner, and they voted in favor of trying.

A number of symbols stand for peace, but I wanted our people to create their own personal ones. To get as close to the idea as possible, I had everyone close his or her eyes and take an imaginary trip. Asking them to picture a place where they had felt safe, I said, "You're alone, away from any commotion. It's very quiet and peaceful. There are pleasant odors, and you feel glad to be alive in God's world. Look around and see if there are any colors that appeal to you or any special sounds. What do you see when you look up? What do you see when you look at the ground around you?"

These words were spoken slowly with pauses. Then I asked the people to open their eyes and invited them to tell where they had "been":

In a pine grove with the whispering of needles on the trees.

Listening to a night owl hooting and sounds of animals going to sleep.

In a boat on the water at Winham Lake.

At Abraham's Falls, listening to the water trickle over the rocks.

In a ripened field of wheat with the heads blowing in the breeze.

Listening to a train way off yonder.

On the hills in southwest Virginia where cattle are grazing.

We talked about all of the places, and as one resident described the scene in southwest Virginia, the rest of us could see it, too — black and white cattle against the green hills. At this point another resident began to quote, "The cattle of a thousand hills are mine." This reassuring line from the Psalms fit so well that it seemed to be the natural theme for our banner. I agreed to bring the necessary materials to the next session.

Having several people who can't move around but who must work together on a table makes fabricating banners difficult. It was therefore necessary to give the people their choice of smaller tasks into which the work had been divided. Even if they could do little physically, they had input and interest in the outcome. In this case two people cut letters I had traced on felt, two others cut out cows and someone cut out green hills, another person glued on letters, hills, etc., one person buttonhole-stitched her cow to a hill and another person made yarn cows' tails.

Mrs. J., with her strong sense of design, made the most suggestions about placement of objects on the banner, most of which were followed. The result looked pleasing to us all.

Christmas Banners

Materials needed:

- 1 & 1/2 yards material such as sailcloth
- Felt for letters
- Glue
- Scissors
- Pieces of cloth, braid for outlining shapes or whatever trim suggests itself

To get into the mood for making Christmas banners, we listened to Christmas recordings and read carols aloud from our hymnals. We closed our eyes, paying attention to the words of the carols rather than singing them. Afterwards, as we talked about the images we had seen, I wrote them down.

The residents mentioned the darkness, the stars, the silence, the way the manger scene looked. One spoke enthusiastically of the nativity and ended by saying, "O it was great and it was wonderful!" That sounded like a phrase for a banner to me, and I commented on it to the group. They agreed and so we began our banner, cutting the words O IT WAS GREAT AND IT WAS WONDERFUL out of white felt. We experimented with placing them on a navy blue field along with several white stars.

As a group discusses and converses I have learned to listen for such statements and phrases and pluck them out. These are uttered spontaneously, and it is much easier to collect original themes this way than to ask point blank for appropriate expressions for a banner. Sometimes I suggest we use one that is right on the mark. If we have a lot of suggestions, I write them down and the group chooses.

After a phrase or words have been selected, I ask which colors they associate with the words. (For banners it is best to choose colors within one color family, with a touch of the complimentary color used as an accent.) I follow their suggestions and bring the colors of cloth they liked to the next session.

More Christmas Banners

Materials:

- Large piece of paper 5 ft. × 3 ft.
- Tissue paper in a variety of colors
- Acrylic polymer gloss medium (thinned to half strength with water)
- Large brushes
- Large black marker
- Smocks or aprons (the tissue-paper colors come off easily on hands and clothing)

It isn't always necessary to use cloth for a banner. Last year we made one from a large piece of heavy white paper (5 ft. 3 ft.) purchased from a local art store.

For this art activity our theme was simply the colors and words of Christmas. We spread our paper the length of one table so eight persons could participate at a time. It didn't matter that some people were working upside down since we were concerned with shapes only. I had bought many colors of tissue paper, which people were invited to tear into strips of various sizes. With a mixture of half acrylic gloss medium and half water we brushed over the tissue paper, causing it to adhere to the white paper and the color to bleed slightly. If two pieces of paper overlap the result is translucent because the paper is thin, and, when joined together by the gloss, a third beautiful color emerges.

We talked about words we like to hear at Christmastime — such as Gloria, Rejoice, Joy, and Alleluia, etc. After the strips of tissue paper had been glued on, we printed these words in large letters randomly with a black marker on the heavy white paper. What a

Christmas Banner

gay looking collage! Like Christmas, if the season suggests certain colors, then it is best to limit choices to harmonious shades within that color family.

One-in-the-Spirit Banner

Materials needed:

- 2 yards muslin
- Remnants of calico
- Blue quilting marker
- Acrylic paint, flesh colored (white, yellow and ocher mixed with rose madder or red)
- Fabric crayons (Pentel)
- Fiberfill batting
- Needles and thread
- Scissors
- Elmer's glue

Active residents in the Hermitage Home enjoy quilting. Although quilting is too difficult for people with limited use of their fingers, we have adapted banners to have a "quiltlike" look. Only a small part has to be actually quilted. Our "One in the Spirit" banner was a successful one of this type. It was also intergenerational, combining the efforts of the Personal Care Unit residents and a year-old baby.

My assistant and I were preparing for class one morning, planning to make a banner out of unbleached muslin and cutouts of the residents' hands. Each resident was to trace the outline of his or her hand onto a piece of calico. The hands would then be cut out and glued to the muslin in some kind of arrangement.

My assistant mentioned that her niece was visiting at her house with the niece's baby, Matthew. Wouldn't it be a fine idea if the residents could see the baby? I agreed. With her usual alacrity, my assistant rushed to the phone, talked to her niece and informed me that Matthew would join us for the class that very morning.

Matthew turned out to be a good-natured baby, barely able to stand in his new red and green tennis shoes. A lot of attention was paid to Matthew as he sat on my assistant's lap at our work table.

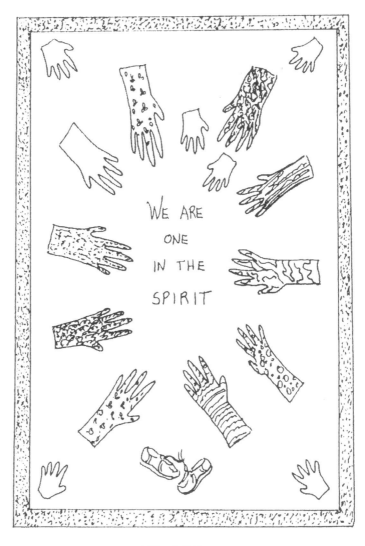

"Hands" Banner

As she and I began tracing the elders' hands, it was only natural to trace Matthew's too. We also traced his tennis shoes and his bare feet. The residents appeared to enjoy having the baby included and laughed at our efforts to divert his attention and draw around his hand quickly before he snatched it away. Together we sang "We

Are One in the Spirit," exemplifying the idea that although we were a group of very young, not so young and old people, we shared a common Christian spirit. During this first session we cut out the outlined calico hands of the residents and glued them onto the cloth.

To the next session my assistant and I brought about ten small calico squares with outlines of Matthew's hands and feet. Each person painted a hand or foot with flesh-colored acrylic paint. Those who were able, put batting between these squares and squares of muslin. They whip stitched the finished squares to the large banner after taking small stitches to outline the hands and feet, creating a defined, three-dimensional effect. This technique of painting on a square of cloth, putting batting and muslin behind it, and stitching through the layers is easier than traditional appliqueing.

For the center of the banner we stitched a square of muslin on which someone had painted in fabric crayon, "One in the Spirit." It was surrounded by large calico hands and then by baby hands and feet. We finished our attractive banner by sewing on borders to match one of the calico materials.

Portrait of Mrs. H.

Goal: To increase the residents' appreciation and knowledge of the use of pastels and portrait painting.

People like to watch others draw and paint. From my experience sketching people on the boardwalk in Atlantic City as a college student, I remember crowds collecting to watch me and my fellow artists as we drew. Through the years I, too, have enjoyed watching demonstrations and learning how painters get certain effects. Thus, when we need a break from our Health Care Center routine, I — or an invited artist — will demonstrate an art medium.

One day in an art therapy class, I was conducting an art appreciation session on the way artists utilize colored chalk or pastels, using the works of Cassatt, Degas and other Impressionists as examples. I had the residents look at the pastel drawings and imagine where they had been done, how many times the model had posed, etc. Carrying my large wooden box of pastels from person to person, I encouraged people to touch the pastels, feel their softness and note the many shades of greens, reds and blues.

About 10 people sat in wheelchairs in a semicircle behind my chair and easel. A young man was to pose for me, and I planned to talk about what I was doing as I worked.

Suddenly Mrs. H., a rather forgetful woman in her 80s, said, "I will be the model." I was very surprised at her volunteering and had not prepared for such a possibility. I didn't know whether she would be able to sit in her wheelchair long enough for me to complete a demonstration. I also didn't know whether I could render a positive drawing or whether I might end up with something ghastly, emphasizing wrinkles and the ravages of age. I had never attempted such a painting before.

Quickly I realized that if I used sand-colored paper and pastels in lighter shades of cream to bring out facial highlights, I could avoid drawing the wrinkles and lines. It would be an impression of her, rather than a full portrait, as I would use as few flesh tones as possible.

Mrs. H. sat in the chair facing me and looked at a point I suggested. Much to my surprise, every time I glanced at her she put a smile on her face and lifted her chin. Even at her age, sitting in a housecoat, she wanted to look her best in her portrait. It seemed to take every ounce of her energy to sit up straight and look pleasant.

I carried on a conversation as I drew, with the group behind me watching every move. This is not easy to do since one's concentration on the drawing is constantly being broken. So it was as much a surprise to me as to the others that I was finally successful in getting a good likeness of Mrs. H., fortunately a pleasing portrayal of an older woman. Since I wasn't able to finish the portrait in one sitting, it was necessary to work on it again. Mrs. H. agreed to wear a dress rather than a housecoat the next time we got together.

I worked on this portrait two additional times for 20-minute periods. In the end I was very pleased and so was she. Surprisingly, the group wanted to watch these additional sessions too. After this experience I did two more pastel drawings at the request of individuals who wanted to give them to relatives.

Since I carry my drawing pen most of the time, I have managed to include other residents casually in my drawings. These are usually more like contour drawings in which the person is recognizable, but without many age lines. I suppose we women are vain, but few of us want to be reminded of our age by the number of lines in our faces.

Self-Portraits

Goal: To create an awareness of one's self, to focus on the sense of touch and to build self-esteem.

Benefit: The residents are reminded of their facial features in a reaffirming, sensory way.

Materials:

- Vine charcoal
- Newsprint or charcoal paper (12" × 18")
- Paper towels

In an institution it is all too easy for individuals to lose their identity in the group, to lose their feeling of uniqueness. It is important to keep before them their identifying qualities that are unlike anyone else's. They need experiences which encourage and nurture the wonder of their differences and which contribute positively to their perception of themselves. Recognizing and accepting physical differences reinforces one's sense of self.

In creating self portraits, the idea is not to produce a handsome product, but to capture some impression of one's self. For this activity, I begin by having participants close their eyes and then stretch their arms and wiggle their fingers. I ask them to touch the top of their heads with their fingertips and slowly feel their hair. Is it wiry? Is it soft and fluffy like cotton? Is it straight or curly? Does it fall onto the forehead or is it pulled back from the face? Do they have a lot of hair?

Then I ask them to bring their fingers down to the forehead and use both hands to feel whether it is rounded, flat, wide or narrow. Does it feel like a high forehead? (Sometimes we have to take a break at this point, because their arms get tired from being held up so long.)

51

Next we come to the eyebrows. (The residents may need help in removing their glasses at this point.) Are they thick with hair, or thin? Do they feel straight, perhaps like one long line across the face, or are they like two small crescents? I ask them to feel the way their eyes are set into the eye sockets. Are they deep set, or does there seem to be no space between the lid and brow, just one piece of skin? Do they droop down at the corners, or end abruptly? Any laugh wrinkles at the edges? Not having any other features to compare with means that the person relies on a subjective idea of how he or she already perceives himself.

The nose is next. What is it like? As the finger is run up and down the bone, is the nose longer or shorter than the eyebrow? Are there any bumps or hooks? What happens at the end of the nose? What about the triangle formed by the nostril and the tip of the nose? Is that wide or narrow? As to the sides of the nose. Are there lines that come down to the mouth?

What are the cheeks like? Do they feel rounded or are the bones very evident under the eyes? I ask them to move their fingers down to the mouth. Is there a little trough between the bottom of the nose and the top of the lips? Maybe the upper lip is straight. I ask them to run their fingertips across the lips and notice how sensitive they are. Does the lower lip come out farther than the upper one? Is it larger or smaller than the upper one? What happens to that line between the lips at the corners of the mouth? Does it curve up or down? Is the mouth wide or tiny? As the fingers travel under the lip, is there an indentation where the lip joins the chin?

What about the chin? Does it feel pointed or lost in skin? Is it wide or small? Taking both hands, they feel the sides of the face and how the hair is connected. Are the ears exposed? Are they small or large when covered by one hand? Does the lobe have much skin on which to hang an earring or is it small?

As they feel the neck, I ask them to think of all the muscles under the skin holding up the head. Are these long or short? With the right hand, they trace the shoulder from the neck to the outer edge of the arm. Does it dip, is the shoulder fat or can the bones be felt easily?

Now that they have felt the areas to be concentrated on, I ask them to open their eyes, encouraging them to remember what they felt as they draw a picture of their face. I tell them that the charcoal will smudge easily if they want to smooth it with their fingers to make shadows or tone, to create a three-dimensional effect. (This exercise might be even more effective in clay than in charcoal.)

Do not expect the participants to draw a very complete portrait. On the other hand, they usually manage to get down on paper something recognizable and characteristic of themselves as individuals.

Help them to discover their uniqueness by what they have drawn. They may laugh but they will recognize that no two drawings are the same and that this is a good thing. Here it can be stressed that just as there are external differences, the ways we perceive things mentally are even more varied. These differences call for acceptance of others' points of view as well as confidence in oneself. Even if people are not capable of carrying out this exercise in pictorial form, it is helpful in sensitizing them to their individuality.

Objects in a Paper Bag

Goal: To heighten the senses and to encourage people to translate tactile feelings into concrete images.

We have had fun with another exercise using charcoal. I put four objects into a brown paper bag and pass it around the group, asking each person to reach inside the bag and touch the items but not to look at them or tell anyone else. I ask them to feel the difference in shape of the two larger objects (perhaps an onion and an orange) and to sense the texture of the smaller ones (like a spool of thread and a thimble). Then they immediately draw what they have just felt. They may draw only wavy lines or arcs—whatever they want to do is fine.

Usually they record the shapes of the orange and onion as being distinctly different from each other. Sometimes I include a stick of chewing gum in the bag and then pass out sticks of gum for everyone to chew as they draw. They have the option of drawing it in any form, already chewed or in stick form.

Besides developing awareness of touch, the paper-bag method can be used to stimulate memories. Put in old-fashioned implements the group is likely to have been familiar with in the past such as dippers for drinking from a water bucket, a darning egg, a small tin shovel used with a sand bucket, a house painting brush, a wooden scrub brush and a large wooden spoon. Again, people are able to feel these items but not to see them.

I ask people to recall a time in the past when they used one of these tools. This provides an opportunity to share with the group their individual experiences involving the same item. We learned, for instance, that Alma had taught in a one-room school. It was the custom for the children to drink out of the water bucket using two different colored dippers, one for the girls and one for the boys.

The group was asked to draw the object they chose since this makes the experience more concrete and the rest of the group focuses on the object. It is not necessary to do an accurate drawing, but to make a shape or form that will suggest the experience.

Pressed Flowers

Goals: To provide an opportunity to work with materials from nature; to heighten awareness of the beauty of natural objects; and to make a product for which residents will have a practical use.

Benefits of medium: It is inexpensive and readily available.

Special requirements: Working with contact paper is difficult and requires the aid of a helper.

Materials:
- A flower press (such as the one pictured below)
- Heavy typing paper
- Clear contact paper
- Glue
- Toothpicks

Working with natural materials is rewarding and satisfying. The beauty of plants, vines, leaves and even weeds recalls the mystery of woods and fields explored and played in during childhood. The seasons are made more vivid and memories stimulated by handling specific flowers and smelling their particular fragrance. The variety of shapes and colors found in a small plot of earth can be mesmerizing. Although fire rules prevent the permanent display of many nature crafts made of flammable materials, they can be brought in for a morning's activity and enjoyed momentarily.

One safe nature craft is pressing flowers and using them in various ways. When I first came to the Hermitage, residents were accustomed to pressing flowers in telephone directories. I found shoeboxes full of old brown-looking flowers that had been preserved by this method.

Later that year on a trip to Germany, I came upon a craft item

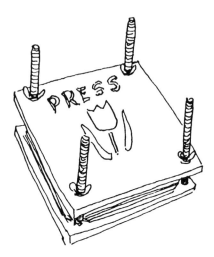

Flower Press

called a Blummen Presse, and realized it was exactly what we needed for the pressing of our flowers. I bought it and began pressing flowers I saw growing in the Black Forest and along the sidewalk in the small village of Neurtingen where we were staying.

Later, at the Hermitage we made more presses like the German one. A volunteer constructed such a large version that the residents could have pressed a chicken if they had wanted to. Here is how to press flowers successfully.

After picking flowers at the peak of their blooming cycle, lay them on a soft paper towel or cleansing tissue between layers of corrugated cardboard squares and stack them between two 1/2" pieces of plywood. The towel absorbs moisture and prevents the marks of the cardboard from being imprinted on the flower. Insert carriage bolts through holes that have been drilled into each of the four corners of the two pieces of plywood, securing the bolts tightly with wing nuts.

After a week or two, remove the bolts and take out the flowers. It is like opening a Christmas package, waiting to see what wonders will be found between the layers of cardboard. The results are particularly exquisite when yellow and white spring flowers such as snowdrops, cowslips, and scilla are used. Other flowers and greenery which do well are pansies, bread and butter flowers, scarlet sage, ferns, mimosa leaves and delicate vines. Many weeds are also dainty and press well.

Sometimes red flowers lose their color, but they can be enhanced by the addition of watercolor paint. To preserve the color of the flowers indefinitely, cover them with clear contact paper.

When pressing flowers in a class, it is nice to have a selection of flowers on hand so the members can choose the flowers and greenery they would like to use. Have each person arrange his or her selection on a cardboard square and initial it before placing it in the press. When the unveiling takes place, it is always interesting to discover how one's own project has fared.

Pressed flowers can be used for stationery, all-occasion cards, small pictures, bookmarks, mobiles, and boxes. A lady in our group places one small flower (covered with a bit of contact paper) instead of her name on the return-address portion of an envelope, thus adding a bit of whimsy to her letter. Bookmarks using 3/4" or 1" ribbon as backing are lovely.

When we make all-occasion cards (usually 4 1/2" × 6 1/2"), I have people arrange the flowers on the paper in a way pleasing to them. Then they apply a drop of glue under each flower. This keeps the flowers from leaping off the page when the clear contact paper is placed over them.

Applying contact paper is difficult for anybody and may be impossible for physically limited people. For this reason I cut the contact paper at least a fourth to a half inch larger than the surface to make it easier to put on. Then the excess is cut off.

To make bookmarks, take a sheet of 8 1/2" × 11" typing paper, arrange flowers in pleasing configurations from top to bottom and apply an 8 1/2" × 11" piece of contact paper. Place a bookmark pattern wherever you wish and trace several on the same page. Some residents may be able to do only the last steps: placing the pattern on the paper, tracing what they want, then cutting the bookmark out. Several bookmarks each may be cut out of one sheet of paper.

To enhance pressed-flower greeting cards, hand lettering may be incorporated, but must be done before the contact paper is applied. At Christmastime our greetings are written with a red or green pen

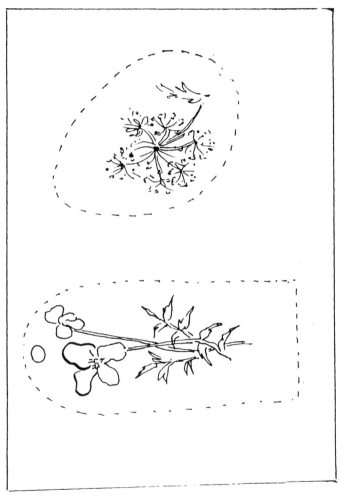

to make the card more personal. For Christmas cards, I try to stick to red flowers and green leaves, a proven way to achieve a seasonal mood. To add a nostalgic touch, holes may be punched on the front of the card and a small ribbon tied through it. This requires some dexterity and may have to be done by the teacher, although the students can punch the holes.

Many times the leader must carry out a significant portion of the project. This is not to ensure a good looking result, but to prevent residents from being frustrated when their disabilities make it impossible for them to execute all parts of a project. I feel that pleasurable crafts should be included in the health care activities even if residents are limited to doing certain aspects. Although they may be unable to do anything requiring dexterity, handicapped residents can make decisions and supervise.

At Eastertime we have placed pressed flowers on heavy pastel-colored paper, covering it with clear contact paper. After tracing egg shapes on the paper and cutting them out, we punched holes in the large end and threaded the eggs on various lengths of string that we then attached to the ceiling. The effect was like a field of beautiful mobile eggs.

Another activity is to fashion pressed flowers into fantasy animals. Residents will need an example to get the idea, but they will soon put together animals with big flowers for the head, leaves for the body, stems or vines for legs and little flowers for feet. Pressed fall leaves lend themselves to more dramatic animals, dragons and winged creatures. Like the flowers, these are held in place by a drop of Elmer's glue applied before they are placed on paper and covered with clear contact paper.

Finally, don't overlook matting and framing the flowers, for they can be exquisite and make a drab activity room look charming. Friends and relatives will be very happy to receive them.

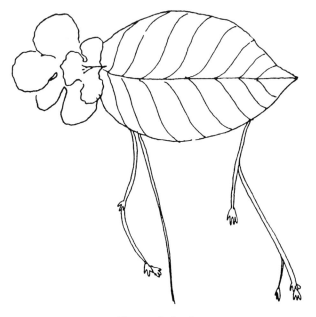

Flower Animal

Parties

Goals: To lift spirits; to celebrate an occasion; to transform the environment from the ordinary to the extraordinary; to expand opportunities for individuals to participate in a group in fresh ways.

Let's have a party!

Everybody loves a party. Spirits soar. Feelings of playfulness, fun, excitement, celebration, deviation from routine, the thrill of not knowing what will happen, visions of Cinderella's ball, Mardi Gras — all are encompassed in the words, "Let's have a party!"

Everybody has gone to a party sometime in his or her life expecting to have a good time. To fulfill that expectation, a change in the environment is needed. It doesn't take much to suggest fun — a few decorations, balloons, crepe paper streamers, soap bubbles, whatever is colorful and different from the daily atmosphere. I have a bubble blower that makes bubbles varying from minute to large. A resident or I may blow them at the beginning of a party, and a feeling of magic and dancing with the wind pervades the group.

A party calls for refreshments. No matter how modest, the food can be enhanced by giving it fanciful names, for instance, "Witches' Revenge" Halloween punch and "Charles Dickens' Favorites" Christmas cookies. I've drunk my share of "Love Potions" and "Mock Champagne" and eaten "Lucky Crackers." Names like these may seem silly, but they help bring on a party spirit.

Don't forget the music and the prizes. Cheerful melodies from "Cabaret," Marches, Scott Joplin tunes, and songs that relate to the theme of the party will do fine. Besides playing recordings of upbeat music, I try to be as positive and good spirited myself as possible. The festive attitude will be contagious. My wearing a costume, doing a little dance step, using dramatic gestures — these help carry the group along with me.

On to the prizes. It's nice when they relate to the theme. For a St. Patrick's party, I used acrylic paint to turn a small basketful of pennies green. Calling them "lucky pennies," I gave them out for almost anything anyone did and made sure that each person had received at least one by the end of the party. At our bazaar party, people got things left over from the bazaar. At the Valentine's party they were given little candy hearts with sayings on them, which the residents read aloud as they received them. Since we were all clowns at the circus party, floppy bows were pinned somewhere to the winner's clothes. And at our wassail party for New Year's, everyone picked up a fortune cookie and read the fortune aloud so we could all share in the fun.

At other parties I have put useful items in the prize basket — combs, emery boards, breath mints, fancy clothespins, Kleenex, pencils, sharpeners, small note pads, candy bars. A lot of old jewelry has been donated to our workshop, so some samples usually find their way into the prize basket. If I have extra time, I wrap the prizes to increase the suspense.

BASEBALL PARTY

Any event can be the occasion for a party. Our retirement home is about a block away from the Richmond baseball stadium. From the Hermitage porch on a summer night, you can hear the crowds cheering for the home team. Since residents in the Personal Care Unit are physically unable to attend a game, we have our own games and celebration.

After singing "Take Me Out to the Ball Game," we divide into two teams. We think of famous sports teams with animals as their symbol of fierceness such as the Los Angeles Rams, Detroit Tigers or Chicago Bears. Choosing a name for their two teams, they decide to become the Hermitage Buffaloes (one member was from Buffalo, NY) and the Hermitage Hound Dogs. I tape signs with the names on them to alternate walls and put boxes on the floor for the four bases. (Jigsaw puzzle boxes work well.)

Then I explain the rules. One team member is to go to bat. If his team can answer the question I ask, he will advance to first base; another question, another base. A question consists of completing a saying like "You can't teach an old dog . . . ?" (new tricks). At least 24 of these axioms are required.

Since many of our people are incapacitated and therefore unable to move easily, I ask active and restless residents (mainly Alzheimer's patients) to be designated hitters and "run" for the others. This works satisfactorily. They put on baseball caps and move from base to base cheered on by their team.

The first time we played this game I went from member to member of the team, asking them to answer questions for the designated hitters. When I saw it was going to make people uncomfortable if they couldn't give an answer, I asked for answers from anyone on the team. This worked better, although one person usually came up with the answer first. After the game we made popcorn in a popper and drank apple juice.

Target Practice

Another game we enjoy is, "Put the Cap on the Head." For this I draw a large picture of a baseball player's head and make small paper hats with numbers on them. The idea is similar to "Pin the Tail on the Donkey" except that the hats have masking tape on the back so they will stick to the picture. It is best to have the drawing taped to the middle of one wall in the room if possible.

One person is led close to the drawing and blindfolded. It is not necessary to turn the person around since this may cause dizziness or a fall. The person who places his or her hat nearest the head wins.

This game may be adapted to any occasion by drawing an animal or a face, leaving off an important part. We have done this with Mona Lisa's smile and Santa Claus's beard. Don't forget to give a prize!

"Bean Bag Toss" is an easy game to set up. People get a chance to exercise their pitching arms by throwing three bean bags at a plywood target with three openings of various sizes. Ours is a painted figure with appropriate openings for the mouth, head, etc.

We have used this target frequently, even with people sitting down as they toss the bean bags.

We have also used it outside. Our administrator was a good sport and stuck his head through one of the holes, allowing the residents to toss a wet sponge at him.

BAZAAR PARTY

The Hermitage and its supporting churches hold a bazaar each November. Afterwards we have a sort of "Thank-God-the-Bazaar-Is-Over" party in which residents and volunteers who worked on it get together to relive the bazaar: the work and effort we put into it, what we liked about it, and what we miscalculated. We recognize those who worked especially hard on a specific part and express appreciation to our chairperson and other leaders. This type of event winds up a bazaar nicely.

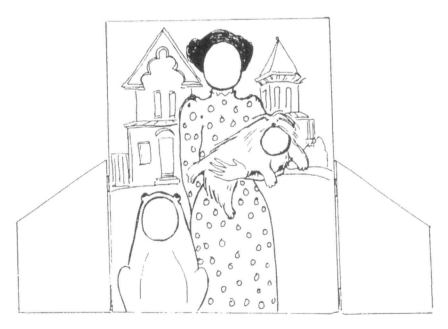

Bean Bag Target

Man-Made Machines

We also play some games. One we enjoyed last year was having four groups each act out a machine with moving parts. Just in case the groups couldn't think in those terms, each was assigned a staff person willing to participate and assist the others in being the moving parts.

To create "washing machine," two people stood with arms locked together behind them moving back and forth while two others encircled them, turning slowly. A "popcorn machine" consisted of several people stooped over in a circle with heads together and another ring of people standing behind, reaching over them and holding hands like a dome over the first group. As the popcorn began to "pop," the inner group stood up straight, flinging their arms upward and then quickly stooping down again. It is very effective when the "popcorn" jumps in a random sequence.

Similar to charades, this game has the added humor of a cooperative effort (with all its possibilities for *un*-coordination) and of sound effects. Since several people are involved, no one person feels he or she has to take responsibility for the results. I have observed reticent people doing imaginative movements in a group, silly things they would never have dared attempt on their own.

Guess My Weight

We have also played a weight guessing game. I begin it by imagining I have lost so much weight working on the bazaar that I must check it. Putting a scale in the middle of the circle, I walk around the circle of people so they can see me as I invite them to guess how much I weigh. A coworker writes down each guess. Afterwards I step on the scale, and one of the residents reads the number. Whoever was closest wins. One or two other people may volunteer to be the subject for another round of guesses.

Since the game is nonthreatening (except for the person whose weight is being guessed!) everyone feels free to participate. Even if they can't see or hear well, everybody enjoys taking a guess. I remember that the person who guessed my weight accurately at the bazaar party was a woman depressed about losing her vision. Her success surprised her and showed that she could function just as well as anyone else at a party.

Cluck Cluck

Before giving our bazaar chairman a memento of the event, we changed the name Mary to her name and sang to her, "Mary, It's a Grand Old Name." (It is helpful to have copies of the words available for everyone.) Afterwards we ate cookies and toasted each other with punch. At parties we do a lot of simple toasting, with residents joining in with warmth and good feelings.

Warm-up

As a loosening up activity at the beginning of a party I lead the group in body movements to music such as "Hokey Poky," "My Aunt Came Back" or "The Chicken." We do bending and stretching exercises, rotating the head, flicking fingers, etc., to energize the body before we play games. "The Chicken" is particularly good as it calls for flapping of arms, movement of hands and wiggling of bodies. Warming up in this fashion prepares the way for easy participation in group games.

Welcome

When people come in the door it is important to greet them as if they were guests in your home. To set the tone of the festivities we often pin a paper flower or name tag on the guests or blow bubbles while escorting them to their seats.

Tried and True

These next games I've used over and over.

Yarn ball toss. First toss a large yarn ball back and forth to members of the group so they get the feel of the ball while music is playing. Then announce that if the music stops while one of them is holding

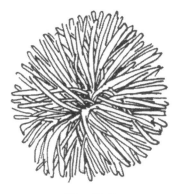

Yarn Ball

the ball he or she must pay the consequences. The person who is "it" takes a folded piece of paper from the hat, opens it and reads aloud what he must do:

- Give the name of your first boyfriend (good for a Valentine's Party).
- Sing the first line of a romantic song.
- Tell about something you're proud of.
- Tell about an embarrassing moment.
- Count four people to the right and say something nice to that person or hug them.
- Act out a job you hate.
- Act out a sport you enjoy.

(These "consequences" can be used more than once during the game.)

Hit the Hat. Have the people sit in a circle around a hat you've placed on the floor. Each person gets a chance to try to toss five clothespins into it. Whoever gets the most into the hat wins.

Follow the leader.

Do you remember this one? Play an old song. The first person to recognize and name the song gets a prize.

Whistle while you eat. Have the people eat a cracker and then whistle as quickly as they can. (Give out only one cracker per person as you wouldn't want anyone to choke.)

Blindfold bag game. Into a bag put different objects such as a hairbrush, clothespin, spool of thread, screwdriver, orange and walnut. Escort someone to a seat in the middle of the room, blindfold the person gently and let him or her pull out one object. While the group watches, the person tries to identify it. When he does so, he receives a prize. Objects should not be too difficult to identify.

Memories. For folks who are mentally competent I put many objects on a tray for them to look at, a variety of things that might have some meaning to them. These might be a Christmas ornament, stuffed animal, hairbrush, key, handkerchief, knife, glove, scissors, etc. I then ask if anything ever happened to them that they associate with an object on the tray.

The tray is passed around so everyone gets a chance to see what is on it. Then it is passed around again for individuals to select one object and tell what their association with it has been. If two people choose the same object, have each tell his or her story. This can take a long time if the group is large, but it is a wonderful way to break down barriers and help people get to know one another.

I used this game on an occasion when I was entertaining a group of people from several foreign countries. Although they had been in meetings together as colleagues, they had not gotten to know very much about each other in a personal way. The game served to bring the group closer together when they shared stories of their association with the objects on the tray.

For instance, one woman from Zambia chose a scarf with spangles sewn to it because it reminded her of the wonderful circus that would appear as if by magic on a spring morning when she was a child. A man from Denmark picked a small brush because it reminded him of cleaning tiny medicine bottles in the pharmacy owned by his father. Others told stories of medals they hadn't won, of baby sisters they had to feed, of a desired item bought with their first paycheck. In a short time these world visitors opened vistas that made them very human and appealing.

ELECTION DAY GAME
IN THE HEALTH CARE CENTER

After singing songs and reading poems with a patriotic theme, sharing information about flags, etc., we imagine what it must feel like to be a candidate for public office. As we consider the confidence a candidate must have in himself to believe he should be elected, we remember promises and claims we have heard various candidates make.

We adapt the "Alphabet Game" to what a candidate could say to get us to vote for him. The game begins with the first person in the circle saying, "Vote for me, I'm *A*-mazing," or "Vote for me, I'm *A*-gainst crime." When we can't think of any more A's, we go on to B's. If the game seems to drag, we move directly from one letter of the alphabet to the next. The words don't need to make sense; in fact, the more nonsensical, the funnier.

HOW WELL DO YOU KNOW YOUR ROOMMATE?

Goal: To increase sensitivity to the feelings and personhood of others.

For use in the Health Care Center, we adapted a popular television game show calling it "The Roommate Game." Three pairs of roommates or friends are asked to volunteer. After one from each pair has left the room, the remaining partners answer questions the way they think their friend would and I write the answers on large cards. Examples:

- If your roommate had to choose a book to read, would she pick a mystery, a romantic novel, or a book for information?
- What is your roommate's favorite color?
- If your roommate has a pain, is it likely to be in her head, in her chest, or in her back?
- If you have a problem, is your roommate likely to give advice, not give advice, or suggest you call someone else?

The answers given by the roommate, written by me on big cards with markers, are kept in her lap. When the partner returns, she is seated next to her roommate and asked the same question. After she answers, her roommate holds up what is on the card and there is either surprise or laughter. Then it is the other roommate's turn to leave the room and a new set of questions are asked and answered in the same manner.

Other subjects include favorite foods, animals, topics of conversation, places to travel, what one reads in the newspaper first, etc. The game is fun and fosters socialization. One drawback is that everyone cannot participate at the same time, but with a large group the leader can offset this by talking to the audience and involving them in the process.

One final word. Anything can lend itself to a party theme: dog days in August, book characters, movies, superstitions, whatever the group has talked about at length. If the leader does some research on the topic and prepares the people a week beforehand, ideas will come and the party cannot help being fun.

Favors — Or Is This Art?

Goals: To provide table favors for 350 people on holidays; to enable residents to feel they have contributed artistically to the community in which they live; and to enrich the meaning of various seasons.

Working in a retirement home with 350 people, I find myself responsible each year for table favors for five holidays: Valentine's Day, Easter, Fourth of July, Thanksgiving and Christmas. It is a large task, but it can be carried out by residents with varying capabilities.

When I first arrived at the Hermitage and went through the experience of making 350 Pilgrims and Indians for Thanksgiving with help from residents, I thought, "This is an awful lot of work — is it really worth the effort? What, after all, is the rationale for making these bits of decoration?" I decided to set down the reasons for and against doing it.

Pros:

1. Making favors is a way for people to work together toward a common goal, resulting in feelings of satisfaction upon completion of a successful group project.
2. When I send out an SOS to the residents for help, people come who usually have no other contact with each other.
3. Residents who think they have no talent like to assist in this special project.
4. A holiday is recognized and commemorated as a time to be celebrated; symbols emphasize the meaning of the season.
5. A festive dining table lifts spirits and causes people to feel, "Somebody cares about me."

Cons:

1. Materials for making favors can be expensive (clothespins, ribbons, pipe cleaners, wooden beads, etc.). Multiply a favor requiring 15 cents worth of material by 350 and the cost is $52.50 for items likely to be discarded after the meal. No doubt that much in food is thrown away at every meal, but the favor represents a week or two of work and is a visual reminder of money expended. Residents feel too guilty to throw away a favor that looks costly.
2. If a favor is complex, the idea of making 350 of them overwhelming, tedious, and a burden on everyone.

The pros outweighed the cons so the next job was to find a simpler, less expensive way of making the favors (at least for most of the holidays).

Thanks to a coworker who copied an expensive favor on the Xerox machine and suggested asking residents to color the copies in with watercolor markers, I overcame my bias toward "coloring within the lines." There was no mistaking the residents' pleasure at coloring the favors and cutting them out.

We developed some drawings which allowed for a choice of colors and which had enough appeal for residents to be enthusiastic. Also, unlike crayons, watercolor markers are not associated with children and so do not carry the stigma of "coloring."

EASTER FAVORS

Butterflies

Materials needed:

- Color photographs of a variety of butterflies
- Watercolor markers
- Scissors
- Stapler
- Access to a copy machine

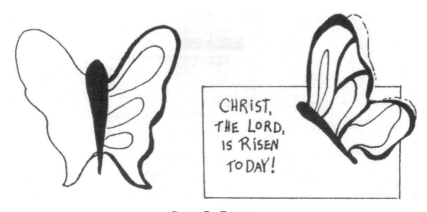

Butterfly Favors

Pictured are some of the favors we have done. The most successful was the series of butterflies drawn from the actual species and Xeroxed. We had reference books out for people to look at while painting the various wing shapes. These were done in every combination of colors and were quite striking. Only one wing was painted; then the butterfly was folded and stapled to a stand-up card on which was printed, "Christ the Lord Is Risen Today."

Each butterfly was different, and on Easter Sunday it looked as though a magnificent array of every kind of butterfly had descended upon the tables in the dining room. The transformation message of Easter was evident.

Easter Hats

Materials needed:

- Scraps of cloth 4" × 4"
- King's liquid starch
- Aluminum foil pie tins
- Small plastic creamer containers
- Waxed paper
- Odds and ends of tiny artificial flowers, ribbons

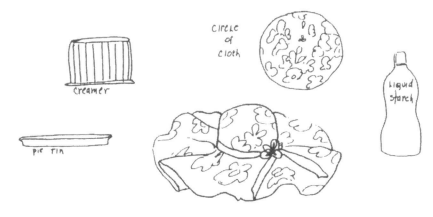

Easter Hat Favors

On one occasion the favors we made for Easter were small flowered hats. Having previously discovered the wonders of liquid starch, particularly King's, we experimented until we came up with a design that worked.

After cutting the material into circles about four inches in diameter, we poured King's liquid starch into an aluminum foil pie tin and dipped the cloth circles into it. Then we draped each piece over a small plastic creamer container (placed on a piece of waxed paper). As the starched material dried overnight, it drooped down a bit over the container to assume the shape of a hat. When the hats were dry, we trimmed them with a bit of ribbon, lace or tiny flowers. We found this an inexpensive favor to make, yet one with a certain charm. (It also put to good use some of the old fabrics in our workshop.)

FOURTH OF JULY FAVORS

Materials needed:

- Boxes of watercolors
- Brushes
- Scissors

- Stapler
- Hole puncher optional

The paper houses we made for Fourth of July favors were fun. I adapted a pattern from the 1906 *Book of Knowledge* similar to patterns found years ago on dull gray cardboard as prizes in boxes of shredded wheat cereal.

The residents painted the houses with watercolors and then cut them out. Staying within the lines wasn't important because the houses were to be cut out anyway. Other staff members and I folded and stapled them together. (A stapler requires too much strength for most of our residents, but they were able to use the hole punch to make holes in the roof, so small American flags that had been donated to us could be inserted.) This was an activity in which all three populations — the Health Care Center, the Personal Care Unit and active residents — could participate. Residents tell me they feel proud when they see something they have helped make being put to practical use.

CHRISTMAS FAVORS

Materials needed:

- Used Christmas cards
- Scissors
- Glue
- Tab pattern

What can we do with boxes of greeting cards and Christmas cards we hate to discard? In the Hermitage workshop many beautiful ones are given to us after they have been enjoyed by the recipient. We recycle these cards as Christmas favors, valentine's, calendars and attention-getters for posters.

Shortly after Thanksgiving we send out a request for people to come to the workshop to make Christmas favors. Residents are able to cut out a silhouette of the outstanding visual feature on the card whether it be a Nativity scene, Wise Man, stocking, house or other

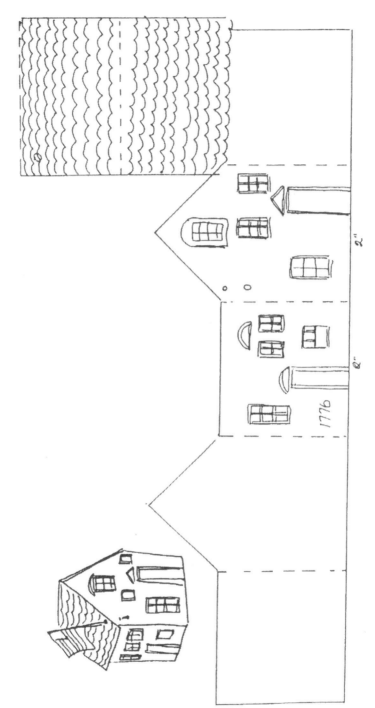

Paper House Favors

feature. Then they cut out tabs and attach them to the back of the silhouettes so they will stand on the table.

This means that some of the favors are small and some are large. But each one is so interesting and lovely that residents are enthusiastic about being involved in an activity giving an attractive second life to cards that would otherwise be discarded.

Here are examples of other holiday favors:

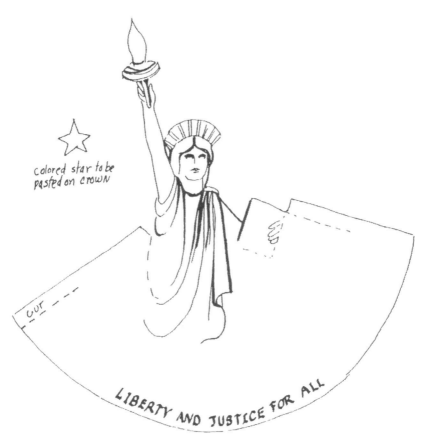

Statue of Liberty Favor

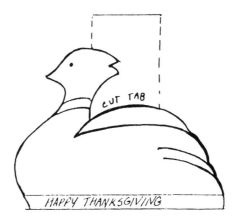

Thanksgiving Duck Favor

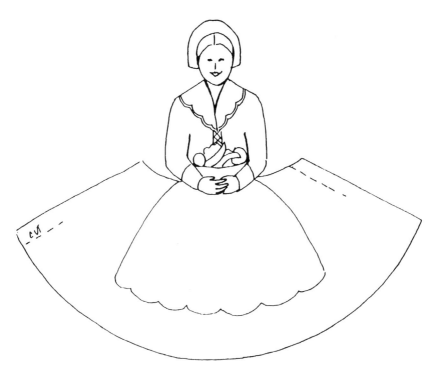

Pilgrim Lady Favor

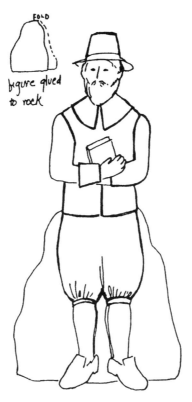

Jamestown Man Favor

Puppetry

As a dramatic art form, puppetry is more common in Europe and Russia than the United States. It can be used for teaching, for entertainment, for communication, and for bringing out feelings along with the imagination and playful qualities of older people. Puppeteers need only tie a piece of rope across a room, throw a curtain over the rope and begin to perform above their stage.

Sometimes persons who are not used to puppets may feel self-conscious "playing with children's toys." Then it is helpful to give a brief history and background of puppetry development. Since ancient days in Egypt, puppets have been used to tell stories, entertain and educate. In fact they were used for the first 1500 years of the Christian Church to dramatize stories of the Old and New Testaments for congregations unable to read.

Puppets were so widely used in Italy to enact the story of the Nativity that they were called "little Marys," or marionettes. Eventually the performers also included the singing of popular songs and nonreligious stories. In fact the performers became so secular that they were banned from the Church by the Council of Trent in the 16th century.

I began using puppetry in the Health Care Center in 1982, at which time we made a small cardboard stage which the residents decorated in Bavarian style. It was made to sit on a table so people in wheel chairs could use it. One of the residents made a little wooden platform, which we cover with a red cloth to set in front of the stage.

We used my own children's puppets, some of which were beautifully made Steiff animals from Germany. Others I had made for the children. I remember in particular a mouse puppet named Mamie, my daughter's constant companion, which I had to repair a couple of times when it wore out. But other than making a few puppets and liking them, I had had little practice with them.

Puppet Stage

My supervisor at the Hermitage, a talented puppeteer, encouraged me to take a class in puppetry conducted by a professor of recreation and an expert in puppet work. So one cold January I embarked upon an intensive two-week puppetry course.

Working both days and evenings, we created three kinds of puppets: sock puppets, hand puppets and complex mouth puppets. Not only did we make puppets, but we had to collaborate with other students on writing a skit to perform for the community on the final night of the course. I would not have believed so much activity and learning could take place in so short a time had I not been involved in it personally. Neither would I have had the confidence or the daring to undertake similar projects later with residents of the Health Care Center and with active residents had I not participated in the course.

There is a certain mystique to puppetry. We were taught to treat our puppets with respect, as though they are little people who should never be hurt or tossed carelessly around. In fact, they, like our art work, are an extension of ourselves. They are a part of our personality that comes forth spontaneously and uncensored.

As soon as I returned from taking the class, my supervisor and I began writing a script. In a short time we were ready to perform for residents and staff. I borrowed a large puppet stage from my church, and we gave our first show. It was so enthusiastically received that our maintenance staff volunteered to build us a stage similar to the one we had borrowed. One of the residents helped measure and sew blue curtains with tiny red flowers to fit it. A great deal of excitement was generated at the prospect of what we could create. After the stage was finished, we began making hand puppets.

Hand puppets lend themselves to a storyteller's approach. One person can narrate the story while others act it out. In this way there is no pressure on people to remember lines or to speak into a microphone as it is not a good idea to put undue stress on people with health problems.

Performing should be done in a casual way, with the understanding that whatever happens is acceptable, that there is no one way to do something. The emphasis is on having a relaxed, enjoyable time. As people become comfortable they become inventive and imaginative. It is a joy to watch them being playful and interacting in refreshing ways.

MAKING HAND PUPPETS

Materials needed: (for the puppet's head; the body may be made by the leader)

- Lower part of a cut-off nylon stocking (for the soft sculpture head)
- Black beads
- Polyester Fiberfill
- Long darning needle
- Double brown thread
- Rubber bands
- Red and black fabric crayons or acrylic paints
- Mohair yarn for hair (grays and browns)
- Very pink pastel chalk

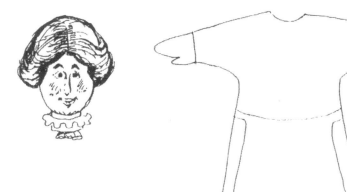

Soft Sculpture Head and Body

Usually the people make their own puppets. For those in the Health Care Center, however, I make the puppets' bodies on my sewing machine, because sewing them by hand has proved unsatisfactory. Health Care residents are able to make soft sculpture heads which they attach to the bodies. They can also participate in the construction of sock puppets.

Making the heads for hand puppets requires these steps:

1. Put the nylon stocking over one of your hands. With your stockinged hand, grasp a big ball of Fiberfill and pull the stocking over it.

2. For now, put a rubber band around the open end of the stocking to hold the Fiberfill inside.

3. Insert a needle at the top of the head and bring it out halfway down on the side you've chosen for the face. Where the needle comes out, make a stitch. This will be the inside corner of the eye and the beginning of the nose.

4. At this point it is helpful to draw the nose, mouth, and eyes with a temporary quilting pen so you have a better idea of what you are trying to do. The pen marks wash off with water.

5. Form the nose by inserting the needle on one side of the nose (which has been drawn like a teardrop) and pushing it through horizontally to the other side. Take one or two stitches, then return the needle to the other side of the nose. Pull the stitches to cause the area in the middle to form a three-dimensional shape. Continue sewing back and forth until the nose is shaped.

6. The edges of the curved mouth should be aligned with the pupils of the eyes. Use running stitches along the mouth line. Take a stitch at one corner of the mouth and bring the needle out where the eyeball should be. Take a stitch and then sew on a bead for the eye. Do the same at the other corner of the mouth.

7. Draw the eyebrows with a black fabric crayon and color the mouth with a red one. Use bright pink pastel chalk for the cheeks.

8. Use gray or brown mohair yarn for hair. Wind the yarn around a piece of cardboard about 5" × 3". With needle and thread the color of the yarn, sew through each strand in the middle of the cardboard to make a part. Clip the yarn in the middle on the under-

side of the cardboard. Arrange the hair on the stocking head and tack it in place.

9. Make a cardboard tube for the neck, to which the head and later the body must be attached. I cut a 1″ ring off a toilet paper roll, reinforce the inside with masking tape and attach the (untied) stocking head to the cardboard with a hot glue gun. I then use my needle to take some stitches where the chin should be, put a dress over the head and sew the dress's neck opening to it. Or put the head over an already existing hand puppet, attaching it securely by sewing the Fiberfilled head (don't use as much Fiberfill) to the cloth one. You need to insert some type of wooden darning egg into the head while you stitch. In a health care center the leader will have to do this part, but active residents are capable of handling the work by themselves.

WORKING WITH MOUTH PUPPETS
(SOCK TYPE)

We have made a number of sock puppets for use by everyone. In working with the Health Care Unit, I encourage each person to select a puppet to which he or she is attracted. A volunteer helper and I will usually assist various individuals in putting the puppets on their hands. I review the motions in how to make the puppet "talk," how to hold the hand upright so the puppet does not lean forward and other basic puppet manipulations.

Frequently the puppet's name has a special meaning to the person who has chosen the name, whether he or she is conscious of the fact or not. The first puppet I made seemed so unusual that I wanted to give her a unique name. I loved the name "Gladys Gillispie," which also happened to be my mother's maiden name. At the time I thought I had selected it for its alliteration and unusualness, but now I know there were deeper reasons.

It is not always necessary for the puppets to be named; sometimes it takes a while for people to get used to their puppet and become fond of it. I think whatever the leader feels comfortable with is important at this point.

As we sit in a circle I ask each person to choose a name for his or her puppet. People have given their puppets names like Ginny-Pooh (a combination of her own name and a baby-sounding suffix), Pistol Pete (named by a man), Mary Smith Jones (by a woman who admires English people), Dish-Rag (by a woman with Alzheimer's disease), Fido (by a woman who is afraid of dogs), Dick (the nickname a woman's father had given her) and Chuck (the name of the woman's husband.)

To remind people that puppets are not merely children's toys, I tell them we are learning the skills of a marvelous profession going back thousands of years. The fact that puppets were used in the Church and remain popular in European countries increases the sense of universality and helps take puppets out of the children's province.

If the people haven't used puppets for a while, it's best to warm up by sitting informally in a circle and converse on a theme. Some possibilities: tolerance, acceptance of people different from ourselves in ideas or beliefs, value judgments, fears and current topics of interest. Or this warm-up may provide an opportunity for someone with a special area of knowledge to tell us about it.

As an example of preparation for a conversation on acceptance, my puppet tells the story of a little boy who was looking for his mother, the most beautiful woman in the world. The setting is another country many years ago. The boy had been part of a gypsy camp always on the move and somehow had become separated from his mother.

He went from village to village looking for her. The leader (another puppet) of each village summoned all the beautiful women for the boy to see, but his mother was never among them. Finally, in the last village, when he had looked at the group of beautiful women and sadly turned away, he spotted in the crowd a bent over old lady with a bundle of twigs on her back. He rushed to her calling, ''Mother! Mother! At last I have found you.''

The ruler of the village was astounded. ''I thought you said your mother is the most beautiful woman in the world.'' The boy looked at the woman, bent over under her load of twigs, and said, ''She is! Can't you see? She is! She *is* the most beautiful woman in the world!''

This starts a discussion of what makes somebody beautiful, likable or lovable. The message of the story is clear, so it becomes a good time for the leader's puppet to be demonstrably loving to all the other puppets in the group, hugging them, and encouraging them to hug each other and talk to each other. Usually a member of the group says something kind or caring that the leader can build on.

One time when I was talking to a cow puppet, it bit me. So I said, "Ouch! That hurts. I'm going to stay away from you. I'm afraid of you."

Then I turned to another puppet and said, "*I'm* afraid of him. What are *you* afraid of?"

One woman as puppet said she was afraid of just about everything. Another puppet replied, "I'm afraid of talking." In that case the puppeteer was a possible Alzheimer's patient who put up a good front socially, but who was afraid to reveal her memory loss by carrying on a conversation. Until then, we didn't know she was aware of her problem or that she *was* afraid of talking.

Sometimes I mention my faults, reminding the group that we all have them. I might ask a puppet to pretend to have a behavior fault that irritates people, like "whining." The rest of us ask why the puppet does that and say how we feel about it. The puppet who whines must put himself in the other person's shoes, and others can practice how to deal with whining. It's fun for everybody to do a little bit of whining together, thus getting a chance to release frustrations by using their voices in a different way. Not everyone will feel like participating fully, but the leader should continue goodnaturedly with the majority who do benefit from such experiences.

I usually end with my puppet hugging or kissing each of the other puppets. Hand puppets can caress another puppet with their arms; mouth puppets, with their mouths. As the leader, my puppet can say, "I love you, Pistol Pete," and convey positive feelings without setting up expectations of a special relationship. If I were to do the same thing without the puppet, that would not be the case.

Other members of the group are able to watch an exchange of affection without feeling excluded or jealous. When it is their turn for an embrace, they can allow their puppet to respond in a free way, saying loving or critical words without the puppeteer being at risk. The residents have the opportunity to give and receive love, something that may not happen often enough in a nursing home.

In most nursing homes, staff is limited, and it is difficult for one leader to spread herself thin enough to give the degree of love each resident needs. Exchanging affection via puppets enables the residents to reach out without raising expectations of a long-term relationship. It is a pleasurable moment.

In a sock-puppet class, I used a Muppet record with Kermit the Frog singing, "It's Not Easy Being Green."[6] I played the song and since some people didn't hear well, I read the words aloud before playing it again. Then I asked each puppet to think of other things that it isn't easy being, and I wrote down their phrases.

The second part of the song switches mood, and Kermit says positive things about being green (the color of spring and the mountains). Each of our puppets did the same.

Since there are long pauses between the phrases in Kermit's song, I thought we could interject our phrases during Kermit's pauses and sing them on one note. We had fun trying, but we couldn't squeeze in all our words. Our activity director, who has a beautiful voice, agreed to help us. She gladly sang Kermit's part of the song, until we could complete our parts during the pauses.

Kermit's Song as Amended

Frog: It's not easy being green . . .

Helen: IT'S NOT EASY TO BE TRUTHFUL

Frog: Having to spend each day the color of the leaves . . .

Sarah: OR BEING A PREACHER'S WIFE

Frog: When I think it could be nicer being red or yellow or gold or something much more colorful like that . . .

Faith: IT'S NOT EASY TO CORRECT YOUR CHILDREN WHEN THEY'RE ALREADY PERFECT

Frog: It's not easy being green . . .

Dorothy: OR BEING CRITICIZED

Frog: It seems you blend in with so many other ordinary things . . .

Roberta: NOT BEING ABLE TO WALK WHEN EVERYONE ELSE CAN

Frog: And people tend to pass you over cause you're not standing out like flashy sparkles in the water or stars in the sky . . .

Jessie: HAVING A BAD COLD AND HAVING TO EAT IN YOUR ROOM . . . AND . . . NOT BEING ABLE TO TALK TO A GUEST

Frog: But green's the color of spring . . .

Jessie: BUT IT'S NICE TO GET A LETTER

Frog: And green can be cool and friendly-like . . .

Sarah: AND NICE TO HAVE PEOPLE ADMIRE YOUR WORK

Frog: And green can be big like a mountain or important like a river or tall like a tree . . .

Roberta: AND NICE COMING TO ART THERAPY AND HAV-ING FUN EVEN WHEN YOU CAN'T DRAW

Frog: When green is all there is to be . . .

Dorothy: IT'S NICE TO HAVE FRIENDS WHO OVERLOOK YOUR FAULTS

Frog: It could make you wonder why . . .

ALL: WE WONDER

Frog: But, why wonder, why wonder . . .

ALL: WHY TRY

Frog: I'm green and it'll do fine, it's beautiful and I think it's what I want to be.

ALL: WE'RE GOD'S GREATEST CREATIONS AND THAT'S WHAT WE WANT TO BE!

It sounded so good we worked on it three times to become used to the words, then taped the modified script accompanied by a pianist. It came as a surprise to see the accompanist playing Kermit's song with tears streaming down her cheeks. When we got to the end, she insisted *everyone* should hear our song.

Since our people have a church background, we use the Bible as a source for stories and parables to dramatize with our puppets. They can provide an introduction to a worship service or Bible study. If we are using puppets during our art class, they can make the story more relevant.

For instance, after the enactment of a parable I will sometimes ask the main puppet character to come back on stage to tell me why he did what he did in the play. This becomes an opportunity for the puppeteer to get deeper into the character and bring it alive for the other participants.

Ecclesiastes 3 lends itself readily to interpretation by two hand puppets. "A time to be born, a time to die, a time to sow and a time to reap" are strong images. We have also tried to portray the story of creation using only animated props. The words in Genesis are paraphrased, and eventually the stage becomes rather crowded with a sun, a moon, plants, mountains, fish, birds, heavens and water all moving around. Crowded or not, it is enchanting to watch.

Puppets can also be used as educational aids by causing poets to come alive. I asked class members to be three poets we had been reading about: Robert Browning, Elizabeth Barrett Browning and Emily Dickinson. When each appeared on the little stage, I inquired how he or she had happened to write a certain poem, and encouraged him to tell a bit about himself. We had studied the lives and character of the poets, but it was more interesting from puppets.

The group was so engrossed in the presentation that I allowed the Robert Browning puppet (as yet unfinished) to appear unclothed. One of the Health Care residents chastised me later. She said from now on people would always laugh when they thought of Robert Browning, because I had complimented him on his poise at being able to appear before an audience without apparel. I felt badly when I realized I had offended her by not treating the Robert Browning puppet with greater respect.

A good time to use puppets is when grandchildren are visiting their grandparents. I have observed children often become inhibited in a group of older people, because so much attention is focused on them that they begin to feel uncomfortable and self-conscious. Using puppets allows them to participate in an activity with their grandparent and takes the intense focus off them personally. They see their grandparent and the Health Care Center in a different way.

Recently a six-year-old boy came to the Health Care Center with his grandmother, a volunteer helper of mine. Immediately attracted to the puppets, he entered into the activity as soon as I passed out the various characters. He caught on quickly how to play his part in the improvised script for "Androcles and the Lion." After the class was over, he helped me carry the puppets back to their room and told me that he would be back at Christmastime, or maybe sooner. It was obvious he enjoyed being there. I thought to myself how nice it was for a child to remember visiting a nursing home as an enjoyable experience and for him to look forward to a return visit. (He has already returned with homemade puppets his mother helped him make after his earlier visit with us.)

Our active residents enjoy performing from the large stage. Lip-syncing to records with several voices is fun and requires little skill beyond timing. We have used such songs as "Daddy Sang Bass," "Blue Moon," "Zippity Doo-Dah" and "Sweet Adeline." Since our record player has the capacity to play records more slowly than the normal 33 speed, we can help listeners hear the words better at this slower pace. We have a good troupe of mouth puppets, most of which we made ourselves.

For our small stage, we clamp lights with reflectors onto two chairs stationed at either side of the table. These shine on the stage and are controlled backstage by a simple rheostat system. The lights are necessary so people with puppets behind the stage can observe through the black curtain what each puppet on stage is doing. The light shining on the black cloth also prevents the audience from seeing the people backstage manipulating the puppets.

Some props and signs become humorous when they seem to appear by themselves. The puppeteer needs to wear a black glove while putting props on stage, holding up signs, etc.

Other members of the Hermitage staff also like to work with puppets, and we have written both humorous and serious scripts. If you don't have time to adapt stories (such as Aesop's Fables) or write your own, I recommend trying some of the many puppet books on the market. Being playful and pretending to be another character may not come easily at first, but with practice one begins to feel comfortable with the medium.

Working with Persons Suffering from Confusion and Memory Loss

Goal: To ensure a successful art experience that will contribute to residents' self-esteem.

Persons suffering from confusion and memory loss need to feel accepted and valued, and to experience enjoyable moments. It is difficult, however, to choose activities that do not remind these people of their limitations. Among the general public, conversation consists of asking each other questions, particularly centering on time, dates and places, all of which forgetful residents cannot recall. Among people with impaired memories, such questions increase the anxiety and confusion they already feel.

From my experience, I feel it's best to tell stories or make statements to which residents may make whatever comments or responses occur to them. If the leader talks about dogs, for instance, members will contribute information about names of dogs they used to have. The leader's description of rituals connected with holidays or with geographic landmarks visited by the leader will usually draw out memories of similar trips. It is best to let people join in when they want to. If one or two people do most of the talking, that's all right, others enjoy listening.

Other group members can be included by the leader's speaking about them: Mrs. W. has brought happiness to many people by the quilts she has made for them; Mrs. H. has visited relatives living in England; Miss M. always has a pencil we can borrow, etc. The more thoroughly the leader knows the residents, the more successful her sessions will be. It cannot be stressed strongly enough that the relationship between leader and residents is the most important factor in these activities; that the leader convey to the resident that she cares about him or her through non-verbal contacts, active listening, or some personally affirming way.

Providing a warm, relaxed atmosphere that is full of good spirit is the first priority. I try to choose activities with an adult character even though they may be simple to execute. If a resident was formerly proficient at sewing or ceramics some skill may remain. If so, the activity may be worth exploring.

Forgetful residents do well within the security of structure. Ordinarily coloring pre-drawn pictures is unacceptable as a creative art form. For a person who can no longer think in abstract terms or form his own picture, however, certain aids are not only acceptable but necessary.

Beautifully drawn, botanically correct wildflowers are available in coloring-book form. Our Personal Care residents enjoy painting them with watercolors. Those who are able, choose the ones they wish to work on; other people for whom that is stressful are simply provided with the materials. Several adult level books of this type are on the market, such as flowers and vegetation with the names in Latin, folk art from different cultures, sea life, etc.

When doing an art activity with residents who have memory problems, it is best to demonstrate with a model for them to look at and refer to. A series of instructions is overwhelming. If the entire class does the work one step at a time, however, more options are open for a variety of art experiences.

I have found that two people working together is a way for both to experience feelings of being effective and helpful. One person may be able to hold paper with holes punched in it while the other threads string through the holes, for example. We have made some very attractive decorations in this way, particulary three-dimensional Christmas trees hung from the chandeliers in the dining room for all the residents to enjoy.

THREE-DIMENSIONAL CHRISTMAS TREES

Materials:

- Red and green construction paper
- Scissors (1 pair for each person)

- Pencils or ballpoint pens that make a dark line
- Patterns for trees (1 for each person)
- Pattern for hearts (1 for each person)
- 6″ pieces of red crochet thread (3 for each person)
- Length of red ribbon or thread for the top of the tree (1 for each person)
- Hole puncher
- Glue

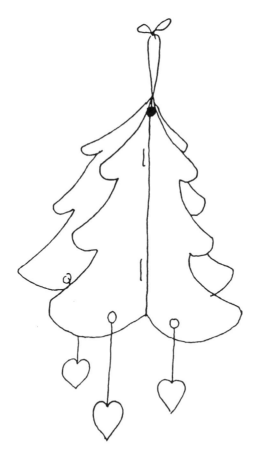

3D Paper Tree

Directions:

- Fold a piece of green construction paper in half lengthwise and trace two trees with a pen or pencil. Cut out.
- The teacher then staples the trees in the middle of the fold (since this requires accuracy).
- Trace and cut six hearts. Place the end of a pre-cut piece of red thread on a red heart, add a drop of glue and put another red heart on top. Make three of these.
- Punch three holes in the bottom of the tree and tie the three pieces of thread through the holes. Punch a hole at the top of the tree, tie red ribbon or thread through it and hang it from a chandelier.

WORKING WITH CLAY FOR PERSONS WITH MEMORY LOSS

Working with clay is a nonthreatening art activity. Given a lump of clay, people often fashion it into a figure and have it say what they want it to. If it looks like something, that's all right; if not, it doesn't matter. They can roll it, pound it, manipulate it, release frustrations, and put it back into a lump without having created anything if they choose. For residents who need to make something specific to feel effective, greenware cleaning and hand-built pots are two possibilities.

Greenware is clay that has been poured into a mold and shaped. Before it can be fired, the rough edges left by the mold must be scraped off with a sharp tool and smoothed with a sponge. Simple pieces without delicate parts can be prepared by forgetful residents. Three-dimensional work, with the task ever evident in front of them, requires less thinking than deciding what color to paint grass or trees.

After the pieces have been fired, the residents can paint them with a glaze medium, a simple procedure. Because a teacher leads the group, people are easily reminded of what they are doing. There is only one color of clear glaze and everybody uses it.

The results are impressive and the residents take pride in what they have accomplished. Naturally many don't remember having done the work, but if they have previously scratched their initials on the bottom of the piece, they recognize the letters and are surprised and pleased.

Hand-built pots, which may be suitable for some residents, are mentioned in the section on clay. People with severe memory loss may not be able to make pots, but you never know what people are capable of unless you try. For instance, a woman who was quite confused did well with a number of pottery and clay projects, because she had worked extensively in that medium before she suffered a memory problem.

Using an Overhead Projector

Goal: To build community; to enrich daily living.

An overhead projector can be fun to use with a group because it enlarges small drawings to room-size proportions when projected on the wall. Just seeing one's name as large as the wall can be a positive experience.

Before starting people on drawings for use with the projector, I sometimes tell them a story, illustrating it with my own drawings. Afterwards I explain that the drawings were done first in pencil on paper, then traced onto sheets of 8 1/2" × 11" acetate with colored pens especially made for an overhead projector and finally covered with a sheet of acetate. It's a very easy process, one I've used with people having a wide variety of mental abilities.

Next we discuss something in the group: a Bible story, song, memories of a particular holiday. If the group has had no experience with a projector, I begin with an exercise I call "small happinesses." This subject is particularly good for people who don't know each other. What a person shares tells something about the person that the other group members can remember. Then too, sharing feelings has a bonding effect.

I begin the session by commenting that life is made up of small happinesses, big happinesses and a lot of anxiety in between. Sometimes we overlook the small happinesses, because we tend to think that our happiness depends on a big event like taking a trip, receiving a gift, or achieving a goal. But in fact each day holds small treasures for us to enjoy.

For instance, when all five of our children were living at home, my husband's "small happiness" was having a clean, dry towel whenever he showered. It was not something he dared take for granted. Personally, I like the smell of a bar of Lux soap, and it is a treat to concentrate on its aroma when I take a bath. Maximum

101

pleasure comes from being aware of the various senses and reveling in the moment.

A record appropriate to play at this time is "Happiness Is . . ." from the musical *You're a Good Man, Charlie Brown.*[7] A small boy sings that happiness is . . . finding your skate key . . . two kinds of ice cream . . . singing a song . . . having a sister . . . getting along. Everything he mentions is small and generally attainable.

When we listen to this song, I ask each person to think of something small in his life that gives him pleasure and to draw it on a piece of paper. After then tracing it onto a 8 1/2" × 11" sheet of acetate overlay, he is to title it and give it to me.

Before people begin drawing, I emphasize that the task is not to see how well they can draw, but to communicate in a visual way something important to them. A shape or form representing something is all that is needed. It is a fact that people are more likely to remember an event if they associate it with a picture rather than reading or hearing about it. This is particularly true of older people.[8]

After collecting all the drawings, I turn out the lights and project the pictures onto the wall. Magnified many times, they are large enough to draw the viewer into them and are more impressive than smaller pictures that cannot be seen by everyone or looked at by the entire group at once. As a participant's picture appears, I invite him or her to tell a little more about the drawing and why he chose to make it. If someone doesn't care to say anything, that's all right because the title is there to help explain. Usually several people happen to share feelings about some of the same experiences, which encourages the group to grow in community and good feelings. At the close of the session I ask the class to look during the coming week for little pleasures to be discussed at the next meeting.

This "small happiness" exercise should be done before the group tackles anything more complex, such as collaborating to tell a story. If they choose to illustrate a song, Bible verse or children's story, there can be musical accompaniment. I find an easy song the group enjoys singing, and we tape it to accompany our pictures. I have also used the projector during a worship service to show individuals' drawings. These need not be complex to be effective.

One November Election Day I was going to merely entertain a class in the Health Care Center. (The constant coming and going of members to the voting booths in another part of the building would prohibit a group activity.) One of my classes had created a "projector show", and I planned to show it several times during the hour to an audience whose makeup would be ever changing.

A large number of people were gathered in the room as I showed the pictures. When the production ended 15 minutes later I expected people to leave but no one did. When I asked why, they told me they were all going to vote in the afternoon!

That left me with 45 minutes to fill. I had brought some acetate and markers so a few individuals at a time could make additional drawings while sitting at a table. This plan was unworkable, because the room was so full of people we couldn't use a table and supplies of acetate and markers were limited. As the group sat there waiting, it became evident I was going to have to improvise something in which the entire group could participate.

We began with general conversation about Election Day elections that had been particularly significant for them, campaigns in which they had been involved, how they felt when their candidate had won or lost, etc.

Eventually we talked about America and important events in our county's history. It occurred to me that if the group contributed ideas symbolizing America, I could draw them directly onto the screen of the overhead projector while they watched them come to life. People mentioned the Statue of Liberty, Thomas Jefferson, the Liberty Bell, inventions of Thomas Jefferson and Thomas Edison, and freedom. When I asked how to draw freedom, responses included "politicians making speeches and promises" and "people going to church." Watching the wall, the audience could slowly see the Statue of Liberty taking form, Thomas Jefferson standing in front of Monticello, the Liberty Bell receiving its crack, Abraham Lincoln splitting a rail, and other scenes.

A positive aspect of this type of demonstration is that it proceeds slowly enough for everyone to catch the images and make comments. Often motion pictures go so fast that residents miss part of the content, not to mention their difficulty understanding the sound track if they have hearing loss.

This occasion turned out to be successful, and my drawing as they watched the wall seemed to fascinate them. I recommend this project if you feel comfortable drawing in front of people. It may take a little practice beforehand, but the group will probably be very patient.

The Poet and the Pudding

Goals: To introduce residents to poetry writing; to enable residents to translate experiences and feelings into word images.

I first heard the poet Kenneth Koch when he came to Richmond in 1977 to speak to a group who worked with the elderly. His book, *"I Never Told Anybody": Teaching Poetry Writing in a Nursing Home"* had just been published. As he read excerpts and answered our questions, I was enthralled.

The idea of approaching poetry writing as he had was new and exciting to me. No need for rhymes, no concentration on meter. The goal seemed to be to capture a moment in time using specific details and involving the senses. I went home that night and wrote my first poem—about one of my clients, a "very proper" old woman who could no longer care for herself, wolfing down food at a fast food restaurant to which I had taken her, obviously starving but still refusing help from me.

After reading *"I Never Told Anybody"* I found that Mr. Koch had also written *Rose, Where Did You Get That Red?*[10] and *Wishes, Lies and Dreams*,[11] both books on teaching poetry writing to children. Following his suggestions I found I could write short, simple poems that didn't rhyme but that managed to convey experiences in a compact form (rather like writing in shorthand).

Later, I took a week-long poetry writing workshop with a poet and instructor from Syracuse University, who gave me additional encouragement to write. I learned to put down a prose description of a happening and condense it into a few lines.

This was the extent of my background when I began sessions in adult homes on writing poetry. It was pretty unpolished stuff, but I found that everyone had a fund of images which could be contributed to a group poem. Some people in the homes were unable to write, and most of them never read books, but they all could describe experiences and share their impressions of beauty and life.

Later when I went to work at the Hermitage I found in the Health Care Center a group of residents who were fond of reading and who felt more comfortable with words than with painting pictures. The two art forms are not that dissimilar, of course. Both deal in images, and both can lift spirits by transporting the person to other worlds when depression threatens. Looking at particular scenes or images evokes a response as does listening to words. Both create an atmosphere different from the one we may be experiencing. I remind people that although we might not be able to travel physically, we can take trips in our minds.

Before the group begins to write, I feel there is a need for preparation of body as well as soul. After doing some limbering up exercises (if you loosen the body, you may also loosen the mind), we sometimes listen to music (pastoral, haunting, folksy, etc.) appropriate to our theme. But we never listen to music while we are actually doing the writing. Often I read poems on our chosen subject as examples of how other people have responded to an experience. If possible, it is also helpful for the group to have something concrete to look at to inspire thoughts about color, comparisons of shapes, etc.

In our writing session we concentrate on describing experiences and recreating images, but not particularly on the pleasurable sound of words themselves. If we focus unduly on the sound, the flow of thought and mood may be broken. When lovely combinations of words emerge, I repeat them several times so the rest of the class can enjoy them. I especially remember "warm winter nights in Waverly," "fourteen stalks of double hollyhocks beside a gas station" and "my name is Sally, I'm a Siamenese." We laughed over the mispronunciation of *Siamese*, but it sounded better in the sentence that way, so we did not correct it.

To convince the class that poems don't have to rhyme, I read selections from Carl Sandburg and Walt Whitman (whose work they probably knew) as well as from William Carlos Williams and Wallace Stevens (with whom they may not be familiar). A wonderful introductory poem is Robert Frost's "The Pasture," with which he begins many of his poetry books. I also bring in tape recordings from the library of poets reading their own work.

An easy way to begin poetry writing is to do Kenneth Koch's exercise on "The most beautiful thing I ever saw." Ask the students to think of something that appealed to them in the past. (I find that if they think it must be the "*most* beautiful" thing they've ever seen, the decision can be overwhelming. It is easier to acknowledge that we've all seen many beautiful things and that they need write about only one of them.)

Next ask them to tell what the appealing thing was and to say specifically what made it beautiful. People learn that the word *beautiful* in itself means nothing, that they must use colors, shapes, specific small details to help other people visualize what they see in their minds. As the thoughts are read aloud people enjoy hearing their own words read as well as learning what others find lovely. They are surprised and pleased that they have begun to write.

Another way to begin is to place on a table in front of people some items that may trigger memory or feeling as they write. For instance, the day we used real fish to make fish prints, it occurred to me it was also an opportunity to write a poem. Smelling and touching the fish as we had, caused the class to think of water and fishing. I encouraged the residents to speak directly to the fish, imagine where it had been and ask questions about its life in the water. They were to include any associations that came to mind if they felt like doing so.

SILVER STREAK

There you are! You silver streak in the water.
Where will you go now, you silver shadow in the blue water?
You put up a battle, didn't you?
But my will to win outlasted yours.
From here it's the frying pan for you
And a fish dinner for me.

—*Alma Lowance*

LITTLE FISH

Little fish with silvery scales
Do you yearn to be once more
In the cold blue water of the lake?
Did you have companions as you swam?
Did the allure of something wiggling
On the end of a line become so strong
That you could not resist it?
You are so beautiful!
You have given us joy
In our efforts to observe
Your symmetry and your shining colors.

— *Kathleen Elmore*

We have written poems around holidays, seasons, and special events. For guidance, I highly recommend reading all of Kenneth Koch's books as well as building a personal library of poetry books. I tend to choose short poems to read aloud or a few verses at a time from longer poems so they have a strong impact. Besides my choosing poems, I question residents about favorite poems they know from memory and we use those too. Since half the Bible is poetry we include Scripture and have even written our own psalms as a result of a class I attended on psalm writing.[12]

After three years of my conducting an introductory course on poetry and collecting the resulting poems, our Hermitage administrator asked me to put together a booklet of the residents' poems. About the same time, I was asked to work with the Activity Coordinator on a resident cookbook. While dividing my time between these two projects, it occurred to me that we could combine them, which would make the cookbook more interesting and assure our poets a wider audience. Thus was born *The Poet and the Pudding*.

Since the book was going to emphasize food, we needed more food poems (although I was going to intersperse beach poems with seafood dishes, seasonal poems with seasonal foods, etc.) Writing about food turned out to be a great deal of fun, since eating is something important in everyone's life.

At the first session I played the record "Food, Glorious Food," a rousing song from the musical *Oliver*, although the words were lost on many older people with hearing disabilities. Residents were told what the words were, and they enjoyed hearing the song a second time. An easily understood recording is Lewis Carroll's poem, "Soup," sung dramatically by Beatrice Lillie.[13] The actress runs the gamut of emotions as she talks about a bowl of soup. After our class heard this recitation of a poem by a prominent writer, they knew that "anything goes" and were ready to get in there and try their hand at food poems.

A basket of vegetables helped set the mood. People chose a favorite vegetable and held it in their hands. I asked them to describe its shape, compare it to something else, write down adjectives that came to mind, recall memories sparked by the vegetable, and look at its particular color. They could talk to it or about it or never even mention its name. Here are some poems from that exercise:

O Carrot, how did you learn
When to grow above the ground
With plumey, waving green branches,
While down in soft, fertile earth
In rich orangey beauty
Grew your succulent nutritious
Gift to "us people."

— *Inez Hatcher*

Thou penetrating globe
With coat of shining hue,
Your flavor adds to stew,
To salad, meat and anything
The cook might choose to do.

— *Hallie Hootman*

Seated by the fire
In comes Mark all bundled
From the cold and golf
Hands full of the gold of persimmons

Of ripe persimmons
For Reva.

—*Reva Gregory*

Needing poems about how it feels to be in the kitchen, I brought
in some aprons for people to look at and said, "Write as though you
are the apron speaking. Imagine what your life would be like as an
apron, when you were put on, what some of the smells would be,
what food would be around you." During this session I learned
something new. Some of these people had had kitchen help and
therefore had worn pretty aprons, not work aprons. A few had never
washed clothes, so their perspective was a little different than I had
anticipated.

AN APRON SPEAKS

Oops, she is too near the stove,
and I'll be scorched.
I was new and crisply starched,
But the grease from chicken frying
Soon made me limp.
When the meal was ready
One careless toss into the pantry
Took care of me until Monday
When Bridget gathered the clothes
For the weekly wash.

—*Alma Lowance*

MY APRON

I have an apron.
When I fried my hamburg cakes
I enjoyed that apron,
so colorful, blue and white.
It kept my dresses clean
And I loved the little thing.

—*Bertha Bowmar*

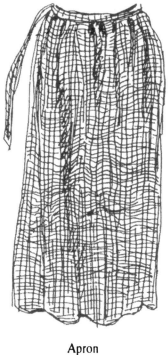

Apron

YESTERYEAR

I wrapped myself around you
When you sat on your mother's lap.
It was on the front porch,
In the evening when the air was cool
That you fell asleep
As you snuggled in the warmth
Of me and your mom!

—Virginia White

On another occasion I served tea and cookies, and we talked about special tea parties we had attended. Everyone could recall a memorable one. A woman wrote about her customary afternoon visit to a tea shop in London. Another remembered meeting regularly with friends in her apartment for afternoon tea at four o'clock.

I asked them to write a description of their drinking tea, the kind of dishes used, what they had had to eat, so all of us could see tea time as it had been for them. Here are more of those poems:

Four Wedgewood cups
On a low table,
One plate of lemon tarts.
It is 4:00 p.m. and tea time
For four ladies who are neighbors.
Suddenly there are three —
Three loud sounds from the door's
Chimes. The ladies come in.
The cozy is removed;
The hot tea seems to stimulate
Conversation.

—*Alma Lowance*

For the final session I used puppets and our small stage. Pretending to be a reporter interviewing people about their lives, I asked certain gregarious participants to take a puppet and go behind the curtain. As I called them, the puppets appeared and answered questions in an interesting way about their lives, the place they came from, what people liked to do there, what I could see if I went there. I also played a recording of John Denver's "Country Roads," because that's where my roots are, and it seemed to apply. Reading "Adelstrop," a poem about a town in England, also fit in well.

Then the participants were instructed to each write a poem. "Tell where you come from, describe something there, and invite someone to come and do something with you there," I said. Here are examples:

JARRATT

I come from an old, old town called Jarratt
In southern Virginia.
There, the fields are flat

And dark and rich.
The village on the Atlantic Coast Line Railroad
Is the center of a well-populated farm community.
There are peanuts growing
And gardens thriving
And fruit trees yielding their produce.
The town was named for a well-known family
Some of whom still live there.

—Kathleen Elmore

PITTSYLVANIA COUNTY

I come from the fertile farm land of
Pittsylvania County.
Join me as we view the lovely fields of tobacco
Ripening in the sun,
Suntanned farmers pulling the leaves and
Tying them in bundles.

Now walk with me to the big white house
in which I was born.
Under the shade of the big sumac trees
We turned the freezer of ice cream.
Later the cool delicious vanilla cream
Was enjoyed by those turning the handle.
What happy memories of my childhood fill my heart
As I revisit this place.

—Virginia White

For the introductory poem to our cookbook we finally settled on
"Come Stroll with Me" by Inez Hatcher, one of our most natural
poets.

COME STROLL WITH ME

Come stroll with me — together we
May wonders find outside my door,
Where Robin, Wren, Thrasher, Thrush

Are building homes in every bush.
And we may sit upon a bench
And talk of hopes, and love and such,
And things beneath and things above —
Until some food we find we crave,
— So back into my kitchen bright.

—Inez Hatcher

Our book ended with a calligram, a poem written in the shape of the object it describes, in this case the fog.

I am the fog. During a heavy summer storm, I hide behind the tall pines when the vapor comes up from the warm earth, I join the vapor, catch an upward breeze and slip like a veil across the mountain top and into the hollow I spread my filmy white, like a bridal train.

ALMA LOWANCE

Calligram

Writing a Christmas Play

Goal: To stimulate creativity through writing and drama; to increase feelings of self-esteem.

Materials:

- *The Christmas Eve Reader*, edited by James Charlton and Barbara Gilson. Doubleday & Co. Inc., Garden City, NY 1977
- "The Sheep Herd," by Sister Mariella (poem)
- Nativity Scripture (Luke 2:1-20)
- Nativity scene with small, individual figures
- Paper and pencils

After we had finished those first poetry-writing sessions, I felt most members of the group were capable of writing a poem if they chose.

Since it was now December, I thought it would be nice to write some Christmas poems. My idea was that each person could select a character who was present on the night of Jesus' birth and write a few lines showing what that character observed or felt.

To help the group overcome feeling it sacrilegious or "presumptuous" to write about biblical characters, I first read "The Sheep Herd," a poem by Sister Mariella, a nun. Then I read passages from Luke about the events of that memorable evening. Last I had them concentrate on the Nativity scene before them, picking up and handling the figures. I asked each person to choose one figure and write a poem or monologue telling what that individual was thinking or feeling about the event. Since three-line Haiku poetry is a simple form in which to convey a feeling, I suggested they each write three lines. (But I encouraged them to take as many lines as they needed to communicate what they wanted to say.)

One woman chose to do the parts of both a sheep and a sheep dog. Another remembered a song about the animals. I initially

117

thought her poem was words of that song but soon found it was her own creation since she was good at rhyming. The woman who chose the shepherd referred to him as the "elder shepherd." Quite a bit of informal talk went on before people settled down to write.

At the end of the class I read some of the poems aloud and we realized what we had was a play! It was an exciting moment and an idea too full of possibilities to lose. I told them I would type it as a script so we could read it the next week. One woman had even written a description of the fields of Bethlehem, which became the introduction. During the week two people wanted to make improvements on their parts and called me into their rooms to listen to the changes. One woman had even written two more pages for her character.

I typed the poems in logical sequence using capital letters for easier reading. Everyone was given a Xeroxed copy of the play with his or her part underlined so he would know when it was his turn to read.

Our practice went so well that we decided to read the play at the Christmas tea for friends and relatives. The members of the group were as proud of their efforts as I was, and I made a point of expressing my enthusiasm.

As we practiced, one woman wanted to make numerous changes in the play, often in parts written by others. I made the mistake of opening up her ideas for discussion. As a result, one woman with a severe speech handicap withdrew because she felt she couldn't do well enough. I learned that in a group effort, it is not good to let anyone correct someone else's work or the writer will lose confidence.

At our Christmas tea we all sat around the Christmas tree and read the play to the assembled families. As two of the writers were ill that day, I read their parts but explained I was only filling in and had not contributed to the script.

The participants were justly pleased with the appreciative response of the audience — so much so that they willingly performed the reading later for two other audiences. As a result of their recognition, they became known as "The Via Players" (after the Via Health Care Center). They looked forward to the performances, taking care with their appearance, using makeup and dressing in their best clothes. The play has been repeated in subsequent years and continues to change as members of the group suggest improvements to their own parts.

THE COMING OF THE CHRIST CHILD

In Bethlehem's field
The night was dark
And there were shepherds
Watching their sheep
But in the sky was one star
Which shone brightly
Giving light to all.

The owner of the inn
Refused to let Mary and Joseph in
So they settled in the barn.
Sounds of the animals were heard . . .

Dog:

I am the dog.
I help the shepherd watch the sheep
And keep them together.
My job is hard
And my day is long.

Sheep:

I am the sheep.
Tired all day from being chased
By the watch dog.

Donkey:

I am the donkey, gray and brown.
I carried his family to Bethlehem town.
In the night a wondrous light
Revealed the birth of the holy child.
So said the donkey, brown and mild.

Cow:

> I am the cow.
> I want to give but I don't know just how.
> I will offer the child some warm milk.

Camel:

> I am a camel, brown and sandy.
> If people must move I will be handy.

Angel:

> I am the announcing angel.
> Hovering over the manger scene
> Coming to look over the Christ child.
> What a beautiful sight to behold —
> the birth of Jesus.

Star:

> When God said, "Go down and shine,"
> I little knew what I would see.
> Shepherds in great fear
> Were running toward the stable.
> Off on the far hills
> Were three kings riding toward the stable.
> Angels sang
> And people worshipped.

An elder shepherd speaks:

> It is strange
> The sheep were restless tonight
> And the sheepdog ran to and fro.
> There seemed to be something mysterious
> In the air, something that could not be explained.
> Everyone was excited and wide awake.
> The reason became real
> When suddenly there was a brilliant light —
> So bright that it was blinding.
> I could hardly see what was causing it.

When I could see again
There was a figure so dazzling and bright,
So bright that I could scarcely refrain
From falling on my face.
He spoke — in strange angelic tones,
Quieting my sheep,
Calling to my sheepdog.
I stood as though transfixed, to hear music
Unbelievably beautiful.
It seemed to be coming from the sky.
When I could hear what the stranger was saying,
These words were distinguished:

"Fear not, shepherds,
For behold, I bring you good tidings!"

Joseph:

I am Joseph,
Alone and insecure,
In a strange place,
Unhappy that this event had to take place
In a stable.
But I am pleased that what the angel said
Was true.
We are pleased to be the parents of Emmanuel.

Wise Man:

I am the wise man
Who came to see the baby
And was so pleased at the beauty
Of the scene before me.
I knew that what
The angels said was true.

Christ Child:

I am the Christ child. I have come.

Laughter

Goal: To provide humorous material that will amuse the residents.

Benefit: Laughter is thought to have healing qualities.

During our year-end evaluation in the Health Care Center, a resident said she hadn't laughed all year. So I decided to brighten the dark days of January and February with sessions devoted to experimenting with various situations people might find humorous.

My rationale for concentrating on laughter came from evidence that laughter is healing, both physically and psychologically. As *Saturday Review* editor Norman Cousins wrote in *Anatomy of an Illness*,[14] a book describing his bout with a serious, painful illness, he discovered that when he laughed, organic changes took place within his body and his health began to improve. Cousins eventually conquered his illness.

A theory advanced in *The Laughter Prescription*[15] by Bill Dana and Lawrence Peter is that the patient tends to focus his mind on the painful area, actually causing more tension and thus pressure on the area. When the person's attention is diverted, the tension eases. During laughter, endorphins, the body's natural painkillers, are released into the system and the patient feels better physically.

The information in these two books seemed reason enough to spend time finding things that would make our residents laugh. (I was aware, however, of friends who had tried Cousins' technique, hoping for a cure, and who had been bitterly disappointed. And I am wary of people recovered from the jaws of death who attribute their cure to one specific remedy.) I also selected movies featuring well-known comedians, read some humorous books and studied clowning.

In the course of my research I discovered three things about laughter: people laugh when something undignified happens to a

123

dignified person; people laugh when they anticipate that one thing will happen, but something totally unexpected happens instead; and the audience must identify with, or have had experience in, the laughable situation for it to have any humorous meaning to them.

I began the first session with a few jokes I considered funny, some Will Rogers quotes and several anecdotes from the *Reader's Digest*. I hoped this material would encourage the people to tell about occasions that had made them laugh.

A woman spoke of a time when she was dining at a fancy restaurant with her brother, an attorney, and two of his clients. Her brother opened the ketchup bottle and shook it on his food. At this point the entire contents squirted onto his plate and all over his shirt, causing the woman to laugh. I pointed out that this was an example of something undignified happening to a dignified person, and that the ketchup's pouring out was also unexpected.

Another woman, someone who had difficulty speaking, attempted to tell us what made her laugh. By listening carefully, I was able to understand that she liked epitaphs. She then quoted a rhyming epitaph other members of the class recognized and helped her with. Rather than regarding epitaphs as depressing, the group was interested enough to pursue this form of humor. At the library I found a book of epitaphs to share with them.

At each of the next four sessions I showed a movie I thought would be amusing. I also asked the class to bring in anything they had read or heard that struck them as humorous. Movies I considered funny starring Laurel and Hardy, Charlie Chaplin or Will Rogers brought forth only a few laughs. I finally realized that the slapstick-type humor of an actor falling all over the place is not funny to people ever fearful of falling. Less overtly rambunctious movies brought no laughter either, although I had chosen actors with whom I knew they were familiar, like W. C. Fields, Mae West and Robert Benchley. Apparently these actors did not portray sympathetic characters. In fact none of the movies I brought caused chuckles, much less hearty laughter.

I researched books and read to the group some pieces from Elton Trueblood's book on Christ's humor, Clarence Day's *Life With Father*, *Light Verse* by Ogden Nash, etc. Nothing received as good a response as the book on epitaphs.

Two of the women thought Bill Dana's scripts "Hose, the Matador" and "Hose, the Deep Sea Diver" were very funny when I read them. I carried this success further by typing scripts for each of them so they could portray Hose and I the interviewer.

Both women had good dramatic timing and, as I asked questions about her life as a matador or as a deep sea diver, each of them gave hilarious answers seriously, as though the unbelievable incidents had actually happened to her. The people listening laughed spontaneously spurring us on to more elaborate delivery.

We found a bullfighter's cape and matador's hat for Mrs. B. and underwater goggles and a breathing hose for Mrs. E. to use for a skit we planned to do at a circus party. But when it was time to perform, I realized I had forgotten the hat. Seeing our need, a woman with severe Parkinson's disease came to our rescue. She asked for some newspapers out of which she quickly helped us fashion a traditional paper soldier's hat, which Mrs. B. wore sideways. This act of kindness indicated how involved the woman was in wanting the show to go on.

Mrs. B. and Mrs. E. enjoyed their comic routine, which we did several times for relatives and once in our assembly hall using the public address system. The two actresses never tired of performing.

Another idea we picked up from *The Laughter Prescription* was to try our hand at writing different endings to the first half of well-known proverbs. As the leader, I wrote the first half of a proverb on a flip chart, and then I asked individuals to give me any ending they thought was funny. We tried several endings and picked the best one:

—A stitch in time saves . . . embarrassment.
—Where there's smoke . . . there's something burning in the oven.
—A friend in need is . . . a friend who wants to borrow from you.
—A bird in the hand . . . is very uncomfortable.

These sayings were not terribly funny, but we enjoyed trying to see how we could make an old bell ring differently. People became more word conscious and willing to say silly things.

We also switched endings and beginnings of proverbs and got a few laughs. For instance: "A rolling stone saves time," "Don't count your chickens where there's smoke." For this exercise I simply typed up a list of proverbs from Bartlett's *Quotations* and Xeroxed a copy for each member of the group. I then cut them apart in the middle, giving everyone a complete set of mixed up beginnings and endings.

During this series on laughter we also tried clowning, a popular movement in the churches that seemed appropriate to explore, especially since the purpose of clowns is to make people laugh. In his book *Clowning in Rome*,[16] spiritual leader Henri J. M. Nouwen says there is "a constant need for clowns . . . who offer comfort, hope and a smile." Clowns show us, by their "useless" behavior, not simply that many of our preoccupations, worries, tensions, and anxieties need a smile, but more importantly that we, too, have white on our faces and that we, too, are called to clown a little.

When I told the art group about an article in a Methodist magazine supporting clowning in the church, residents expressed negative feelings toward linking this kind of behavior with religious institutions. I said I understood how they could think masks and clowns didn't belong there but asked them to keep an open mind. They had no objections to learning about clowns.

We discovered that clowns are not ordinary people but appear to be from another world; they communicate without words and do not take themselves seriously; they are vulnerable, open to others; they may appear to be misfits in society, set apart from the majority; they are sometimes called "fools for God" (I Cor. 4:10); and they suggest the absurdity of life.

At the library I found a technical book on clowning and we did exercises suggested by the author. We learned to move in slow motion to exaggerate an action. We also practiced doing a "double take" in which we looked at an object, slowly turned our heads away from it, then jerked our heads around to focus on it again with an "I don't believe it!" look of astonishment on our faces.

Another thing clowns do is to use an object in an unexpected way. We made a game of pretending a bunch of plastic flowers was something else and having onlookers guess what we were pretending. My group was surprisingly innovative. B. pretended to eat the flowers and exaggeratedly spit out the seeds; M. acted as though they were a clothes brush as she dusted herself off; K. pretended they were a pillow and did such an excellent job of resting her head and snoring that I almost believed she had gone to sleep.

After working on clowning for three sessions, we decided a circus party should be the culmination of our attempts. We made hats for it, and put a little makeup on those who attended. The room was decorated with lions and tigers in cages. I wore a ringmaster's costume and other members of the staff dressed as clowns. We reminded the group that there is a bit of the clown in everyone as we played nonsensical games (some of those listed in the party section).

Our art group demonstrated the use of a common object in an uncommon way, as clowns do, while the audience guessed what it had become. For our beanbag toss, I had made a large plywood target, a picture of a woman with a dog in her arms and an enormous frog beside her. Openings for the beanbag to go through were in the woman's face, the dog's head and the frog's mouth.

Our residents enjoyed these sessions on laughter but I still haven't discovered a way to make frail, older people laugh heartily.

Looking Back, Looking Ahead

Goals: To give the group an opportunity to think about expanding their ability to express themselves in a creative way; to exhibit concrete evidence of the past year's accomplishments; to give the leader an opportunity to receive resident input in planning for the year ahead.

At the end of a year or an experience, it is important to take time to reflect on it, to have "closure." For example, when paintings have been finished in an art class, it is helpful to put them up on a wall, so they can be on view for a while and so the group can see what they have accomplished and then let go of the experience. Other classes need acknowledgment of their value and an honest appraisal as well.

It sometimes happens in a nursing home that art classes are conducted on a week-to-week basis with something different at every session. There is little continuity from one class to the other, no beginning, middle, or end. Classes like this may be fine in themselves, but the teacher and participants have no sense of where they are progressing or what they have accomplished. The underlying feeling is that the classes aren't going anywhere, so the work is not taken very seriously. Leaders following this pattern are likely to burn out. Since I have done it both ways, I highly recommend taking a subject or theme and exploring it for several weeks.

The natural time to evaluate activities and reflect upon them is at the end of a year. We do this New Year's week and set the next year's goals together. I think there is a tendency to avoid this type of discussion in a health care center, because it is painful for residents to accept being there. The unspoken thought is that they are there waiting to die. This thought however is more often on the minds of outsiders than it is on those of residents who have a variety of interests. It may also be depressing for residents to admit they are

129

going to be there in the future. So patients and staff avoid the subject of goal setting.

My belief (and it certainly isn't original) is that people feel better
if they face what they fear. When they talk about the feared thing
and see themselves as able to survive, they can go on to recognize
what strengths they possess to cope with it. They can use those
strengths to enhance their own well-being. Even though they perceive themselves as weak and dependent, they are in fact strong or
they wouldn't have overcome obstacles in the past and lived as long
as they have.

Since people may remain in a health care center two to seven
years, it is worthwhile making that time one of quality. One woman
remarked to me, "I'm glad I came to the Hermitage. Otherwise I
would never have painted again."

For the evaluation, I bring in samples of the year's various projects and experiences to stimulate memories of our art sessions.
Sometimes the array is impressive, and we cannot help feeling we
have accomplished a great deal. To see concrete materials as evidence of the year's work – puppets, painting, clay sculptures, poems – is exciting. Not only does the class feel good about the whole
situation, but I do too!

Inevitably some things have not worked well in the past year, and
we talk about that, too. But as we let go of the past, we come up
with new ideas from the old. During the evaluation, mention is
often made of memorable events that took place in other groups,
and we learn from those as well.

If the leader hasn't done an evaluation before, it can appear
threatening because of the fear that people will say nothing was
successful – or will not be willing to set goals. Such a discussion is
unpredictable but beneficial, because the leader learns how his or
her program was perceived and can now make changes to better
serve the residents.

I have also done yearly evaluations in the Personal Care Unit,
where many people are forgetful yet able to respond to the examples
of work we have done and make comments. Sometimes they mention places they like. That gives me an idea of what appeals to them
so I can incorporate it into a future program.

From our discussions may come suggestions that pertain to areas outside my domain, in which case I pass them on to the proper departments. For instance, several people in one of my classes voiced concerns about feeling trapped, nervous and unable to sit still. I mentioned this to the activity director and volunteer services, and the information helped them design programs for these particular residents.

People need frequent opportunities to express their thoughts and desires so they will feel they can make an impact on their environment. Sometimes changes occur as a result of patients' speaking out. We developed access to a bus as a result of a discussion in which people voiced a desire to go outside. Ironically, the woman who most wanted to go out for a ride went one time and could not be persuaded to go again. The reality of the situation did not live up to her expectations, but it was apparent others benefitted from the dream she had expressed.

Evaluation is also an opportunity to help people set realistic expectations by limiting them to goals that can be achieved within the walls of the health care center. One New Year's Day when we were talking about what we would like to achieve, Ms. M. said that she thought people make a mistake in writing resolutions that are too grand ever to be kept. She realized she herself had done that, such as thinking she would drive a car again, move into an apartment on her own, and get a job. A more realistic resolution for her would be to learn to type with one hand since her other hand and the lower part of her body were paralyzed. This resolution seemed possible since a lot of her writing had been published in the past.

Other goals included being able to hang up a dress on a hanger, singing a solo, and wanting to laugh again (voiced by a woman who hadn't laughed out loud all year). Fears were also discussed, particularly the fear of falling, a realistic anxiety since everyone had fallen, with sometimes serious consequences. We talked about what they would do if they fell, how they could cope with whatever happened to them, how they had handled problems in the past. It was a good session with everyone participating.

In an "ending" discussion like this there is a feeling of sharing. The group is brought closer together by their common emotions and vulnerabilities. And I receive suggestions for the coming year and a feeling that my work has been worthwhile.

The Two-Way Street

Most of the art work described in this book was done by people in our Health Care Center or by people who needed assistance in daily living. They ranged in age from 75 to 90. Few had ever received training in the arts, and few had developed skills in these areas. They took part in whatever activities were offered daily, and joined my groups on the days we were making art work.

Many of the artists had physical problems that required medical attention and all suffered from one type or another of psychological loss: loss of family, productive work, private home, independence, mental agility. All of these had been important contributors to a sense of identity and self-esteem in their younger days.

Because of these factors my primary goal was to provide art experiences to help increase self-esteem and nurture a sense of identity. The art forms became vehicles to stimulate imaginations, to unlock playfulness, and to enable the artist to communicate a personal vision.

Before successful art expression could take place, however, I needed to establish a trusting relationship with my students. Before introducing a project, I took the time to make contact with each person in the group in order to reaffirm his or her presence, often through touch. (A volunteer always shared in this exercise and was there to help in the event of a crisis or in case a participant had to leave.)

The students seemed to know that I cared about them and valued their work. Being a person who responds to the art elements of almost everything in the world, I could truly appreciate the marks they made, the weight of a line, the bits and pieces of color, the blurred image. I found their efforts to be invigorating.

Since I believed that everyone could communicate through some form of art work, the challenge for me was to find the particular

133

opportunity that would best allow an individual to feel effective, to discover his own "art voice." When that happened I was elated.

The relationship worked both ways — I was stimulated by the artists and they in turn learned from and were encouraged by me. As I continued to take art classes, I learned new directions that I could adapt and pass on to the residents.

For example, I learned to use the word "restate" when I wasn't happy with a first pencil line I had drawn. I would then go over it again with a better line. My students quickly picked up on this idea and executed some quite interesting drawings (after they stopped erasing, relaxed and "restated" a variety of lines until they got the images they wanted).

I enjoy doing art work and interacting with people doing art work. In such a relationship it isn't essential to exhibit a jovial, animated personality, which sometimes makes residents feel overwhelmed, but it is important that the leader of the group be able to reach out to the others in a way that is comfortable for her. Her self-confidence and her enthusiasm for her art sessions contribute to an atmosphere of anticipation which seems to heighten the senses of group members. I do not mean to suggest that everyone will respond positively; some will choose to simply sit and watch. That is why the leader must have confidence in the value of her art projects so that she does not take as a personal rejection the refusal of certain individuals to participate. To those people she needs to communicate her care and concern for their well-being.

Literature on working with those of advanced age shows how popular it is to do life reviews and reminiscences. When I began leading groups of older people in art activities, I, too, devoted much time to drawing the milestones of life, recalling holiday customs, and re-creating work done in the past. But I found that this path was not a good one to continue along for any length of time. It began to feel as though only the past was significant, and the present held no promise. This led me to discard the past as the main focus and to begin engaging people in new experiences relevant to today's world.

My years in a retirement community, helping residents to express themselves through art activities, have given me the opportunity to observe the behavior and attitudes of older people. I have recognized a common pattern in those who are happiest. They are those who have let go of the past and do not dwell on events of long ago. Whether that past included numerous achievements or held painful memories, the happier people don't spend much time reliving old experiences; their curiosity centers on what they see around them and what is happening now. This interest makes it possible for them to relate to others with empathy, and to experience control over their lives. As a consequence of this way of functioning, they receive positive responses from the community in which they live, where they are regarded as vital and alive.

When I look at these people who are learning and growing just as I am, I realize that there is not much difference between us. We are in this endeavor together, sharing our knowledge and experience with each other. I enjoy the association immensely and hope that I remember what they have taught me when the time comes for me to let them go.

End Notes

1. Bruno Bettelheim, *The Informed Heart* (New York: Macmillan, 1960; Avon Books) 259.

2. Bettelheim, 259.

3. *Ultimate Thunder*, Syntonic Research, Inc., 175 Fifth Ave., New York, NY 10010 (Cassette #SC99002).

4. "The Eagle and the Hawk" (Denver-Taylor). John Denver's Greatest Hits. RCA Victor, 1973.

5. Peter, Paul & Mary. Warner Bros.-Seven Arts Records. WS1785.

6. The Muppet Show. *Bein' Green* (Reposo) 1977 Jim Henson Associates, Inc., 1977 Arista Records, Inc., 6 West 57th St., New York, NY 10019.

7. "Happiness" from *You're A Good Man Charlie Brown*. Crickettone Chorus & Orchestra featuring Ron Marhsall, Cricket Records. HAPPYTIME 8-16 43rd Ave., L.I.C., New York 10001.

8. "Elderly Retain Information in Picture Format," *Morgantown Post*, Sept. 1985. Quoting Dr. Denise Park, University of North Carolina, Charlotte, NC. ". . . the memory for pictures does not appear to have as substantial a decline as the memory for verbal material."

9. Kenneth Koch, *"I Never Told Anybody": Teaching Poetry Writing in a Nursing Home* (New York: Vintage Books, 1978).

10 Kenneth Koch, *Rose, Where Did You Get That Red?, Teaching Great Poetry to Children* (New York: Vintage Books, 1974).

11. Kenneth Koch, *Wishes, Lies and Dreams, Teaching Children to Write Poetry* (New York: Vintage Books, 1970).

12. Donald L. Griggs, *Praying and Teaching the Psalms* (Nashville: Abingdon Press, 1984).

13. *Nonsense Verse of Carroll and Lear*. Beatrice Lillie singing "Soup." Caedmon, 19995 Broadway, New York 10023.

14. Norman Cousins, *Anatomy of an Illness* (W.W. Norton & Co., Inc., 1979).

15. Lawrence J. Peter and Bill Dana, *The Laughter Prescription*, "The Tools of Humor and How to Use Them" (New York: Ballantine Books, 1982), pp. 8 & 9.

16. Henri J. M. Nouwen, *Clowning in Rome* (Garden City, NY: Image Books, 1979), p. 110.

Printed and bound by CPI Group (UK) Ltd, Croydon, CR0 4YY

17/10/2024

01775687-0003